The Experience of Introversion

To my parents

KJS

To my wife and children

IEA

The Experience of Introversion
An integration of phenomenological, empirical, and Jungian approaches

Kenneth Joel Shapiro, *Bates College*, and
Irving E. Alexander, *Duke University*

Duke University Press   Durham, N.C.   1975 0190762

© 1975, Duke University Press
L.C.C. card no. 74-83142
I.S.B.N. 0-8223-0328-0
Printed in the United States
of America

Contents

Preface

This essay has a dual purpose. It is an attempt to bring current and newly developing phenomenological approaches to personality into a constructive union with traditional empirical methods. To illustrate the potential fruitfulness of such a marriage, we have chosen a particularly recalcitrant problem in psychology, introversion. The second purpose is to reexamine this classic and pervasive concept in personality in light of our joint methodology.

Introversion, along with its counterpart extraversion, has enjoyed a long if checkered career in academic psychology. At some moments it has occupied center stage in the personality literature, while at others it has faded into the scenery only to emerge again slightly recast. The importance of the role introversion and its derivatives have played in the study of individual differences and in the field of personality more generally has not often been recognized. It has in addition been a major vehicle for a number of methodological advances in personality such as factor analysis and Q sort. Outside of psychology, of course, "introversion" and "extraversion" have become part of the language. With only mild exaggeration, we may state that we are as likely to understand the difference between John and Mary in these terms as through the fact of their respective sexes.

Still other reasons for the choice of introversion will unfold in the exposition. For now it is a fitting focus because of the following proposition which we eventually shall justify and substantiate. While introversion clearly refers to a recognizable, readily ascribable, and fully-fleshed phenomenon of personality, the approaches to it in the field of personality leave it notably desiccated and reduced on the whole, and disparate and disjointed in its parts. An exception exists in the writings of C. G. Jung which, as we shall see, have their special limitations.

This problem in personality thus invites the integrated approach that we shall develop and illustrate by application in what follows. The experiential part of this approach has its basis in phenomenological psychology and, to a lesser extent, in existential analysis.* A

*The term "phenomenology" in the present manuscript refers to a method and a set of ideas about experience originating in the writings of Husserl. (See H. Spiegelberg's two volume work for a history of the development of these ideas from Husserl to the present [1969]). We make a distinction between this usage and the broader and looser usage by,

background and context will be given in the general introduction to follow. Some of the assumptions and constitutive features, and an investigatory stance implicit in them, will be described more fully in chapter 3. For the moment the approach contains a particular stance to the theoretical material on introversion, some empirical data, and the phenomenon itself—all taken together. In this investigation there is an attempt to create a dialogue among these three sections by inhabiting them in turn, by living through them as experienced, by letting them prereflectively point to and advance toward the essential experience of the phenomenon. The goal of the investigation is a formulation of the phenomenon in descriptive experiential terms. In terms of its view of the general object of its study, the person, this approach begins with man as an experiencing being who both constitutes and is constituted by a world; who necessarily both creates a world (invests it with meaning); and yet for whom it is always "already there" (Merleau-Ponty, 1962, p. xvii) since he is inextricably inserted in it, threaded to it, and has his being in it.

The essay is in four chapters. The first two each present a set of guidelines which are then employed in the kind of dialogue we have mentioned and will further describe. The first deals with and stays within theoretical considerations. It is an effort to elucidate Jung's concept or concepts of introversion by reexamining his writings on the subject. The second chapter reports some empirical data on introversion which were gathered by use of a projective technique, the Thematic Apperception Test; results are in the form of a construct of introversion. The third chapter presents an integrated methodology, and the final chapter is an experiential formulation of introversion based on the theoretical and empirical guidelines and on recourse to the target phenomenon itself as experienced.

Our hope and intent is that the volume will be read in its entirety as a presentation of a promising orientation to personality. As such, it demonstrates a method whereby traditionally gathered empirical data and clinically derived theory can be integrated and enlivened through an experiential stance, and it offers a fresh attempt at reintroducing introversion, one of Jung's seminal insights, into psychology. We have organized the book, however, so that the reader

among others, psychologists such as Snygg and Combs, Lewin, and Rogers as an equivalent to any person- or subject-oriented psychology, to the phenomenal field, to a perceptual frame of reference, etc. See Kockelmans (1971) for a discussion of these distinctions.

may proceed selectively according to his bent. A casual reader seeking greater understanding of his two roommates or of his relation with his wife may skip directly to the "experience of introversion" section in chapter 4. The student of Jung may want to focus on the explication of Jung's theoretical writings in chapter 1 and on the experiential formulation in chapter 4. The more experimentally oriented student of personality may want to skim the Jungian theoretical considerations and focus on the empirical work in chapter 2. The reader with special interest in or curiosity about phenomenological psychology may wish to read the summary points of the first two chapters and spend the major part of his time with the third and fourth chapters.

The manuscript represents for its authors the results of a fruitful and enjoyable collaboration over a number of years. It began when the senior author during the course of his graduate study became involved in an informal research seminar led by the junior author. The focus of that seminar was a critical discussion of Jungian concepts with an avowed aim of examining them empirically. As it turned out, the typology aroused most interest since it appeared to be most amenable to study by objective methods. Various members of the group embarked on specific research projects.

The work to be reported here had a particular history in that it went far beyond our original plans. As the critical and empirical aspects of the work progressed, the senior author began to read broadly in the field of phenomenology and was excited by the prospect of linking this approach to our conceptual framework in concepts we were examining. An early marking point in this progression was the doctoral dissertation of the senior author. Adopting this elaboration of the task was not a simple matter. It involved ultimately the reversal of roles. The teacher became the student and vice versa. Looking back, it now seems we went through two distinct cycles in our relationship, both beginning with a student-teacher phase and ending as colleagues and collaborators. We have learned much from each other, not only intellectually but personally. To examine the experiential aspects of introversion involved a sharing of life experiences which was both stimulating and rewarding.

But we were not alone in this enterprise and wish to express our gratitude to the various people who contributed to our thinking. The members of the original seminar, David Cook, Steve Bieler, Ron Ginsburg, helped to start us on our way; David McClelland of Harvard University and Harold Schiffman of Duke University were sources of support during the empirical phase. For KJS, Tony Cowgell of Duke provided a critical ear, and Andrea Shapiro offered a nurturant soul throughout. For IEA, these same functions for more than twenty-five years have been performed by Silvan Tomkins of Livingston College, Rutgers University.

The Experience of Introversion

Introduction

There have been a number of "calls" in psychology in recent years which issue from a common question regarding the proper character or identity of psychology and the social sciences in the world today. A very particular call has been for the application of experiential approaches to problems in psychology.

More precisely, there has been a plea for applying approaches derived from phenomenology and existentialism. Several contributors to Wann's *Behaviorism and Phenomenology: Contrasting Bases for Modern Psychology* (1964), notably R. MacLeod and S. Koch, sounded this appeal. Similarly, a number of popular anthologies published in this general area impart this message, including those of May et al. (1958) and Ruitenbeek (1962). Since then, Gendlin (1962), combining insights from the work of Husserl, Merleau-Ponty, and Sartre with his knowledge of psychotherapy, has undertaken a "philosophical treatise" in an effort to carve out and to make accessible a working concept of experience or "experiencing." This effort is presented both as a new departure and as a rapprochement, a synthesis with traditional psychology. Gendlin explains the need for and offers a "new type of concept . . . that can directly refer to experiencing" (p. 21). At the same time he argues that this type of concept and a method employing it can be integrated with traditional positivistic or objectivistic modes of inquiry. Van Kaam (1966) has also attempted to construct a theory in more global terms which synthesizes existential phenomenology with traditional approaches. Both of these writers present applications of their views. (See, for example, Gendlin's work on "focusing" [1969] and Van Kaam's "application of the phenomenological method" to the "experience of feeling really understood" [1966, pp. 294–329].)

In addition to these applications there have been few others (see particularly Giorgi et al., 1971). For the most part the call for experiential approaches to problems in psychology has heard in response only echoes of itself. This lack is particularly striking given the generally acknowledged need for enlarging the foundations, the methods, and the subject matter of the field, some threads of which we shall sketch briefly. Our work follows the lead suggested by Gendlin. It is an extended application of a phenomenological approach integrated with more traditional objectivistic approaches. We

3

shall, however, differentiate our effort more precisely from other applications of experiential approaches at a later point. First, we shall provide a wider perspective for what we have done.

In the late 1950s, C. P. Snow in his *Two Cultures and the Scientific Revolution* proposed the thesis that a cleavage has developed between the natural sciences and the humanities with the recent acceleration in growth of the former. A debate which has ensued between the two combatants has been hampered by the fact that the issue debated concerns their inability to speak to one another. For this reason, among others, the debate, mediated by a recent intruder, has continued into the present. The social sciences, as their name suggests, sit between the natural sciences and the humanities borrowing content from the latter and adopting from the former its methods, philosophy, and objectives. In its social science aspects psychology has been struggling to work out its identity. Its dominant identification has been with the natural sciences, especially with the method of the physical sciences at a time when that method was staunchly positivistic and objective.

However, several instances of growing maturity are evident, including a move toward independence on the one hand and attempts at a fruitful integration of the separated parents on the other. We are, of course, really too close both in time and in investment to accurately describe, let alone appraise, these developments. But we shall disentangle a few threads to locate further the present work and, too, by giving our view of these developments, to state, implicitly, a direction in which we would like to see psychology continue to move.

Enlarging the domain of psychology

One trend is toward enlarging the circle of topics which the field can and will investigate. There is, for example, an increasing willingness to tackle phenomena which might be called supernormal in that they are at the upper reaches of human capability and potential. A brief survey of such topics indicates an awakening concern with both "how to be one's self" and "how to be with another person" in the most productive and fulfilling ways. Within the former consideration, such topics as creativity (Wallach, 1965; Koestler, 1967), altered and heightened states of consciousness (Tart, 1969), "focusing" (Gendlin, 1969), internal focus (Singer, 1966), "peak experience" (Maslow,

1962), loneliness (Moustakas, 1961) are among those studied. Within the latter framework, studies of different kinds of relatedness and interpersonal relations such as the encounter (May et al., 1967; Perls, 1969; and others), the I-Thou relation (Buber, 1958), authenticity (Bugental, 1965), open-mindedness (Rokeach, 1960), and the "allocentric" mode of perceptual relatedness (Schachtel, 1959) are considered.

A clear characteristic of such a broadened area is that the phenomena under investigation are now more experiential than formerly. While occasionally they may be measured by nonexperiential indices or operations, behavioral or physiological, target phenomena such as different states of awareness, various modes of relating to the other, and the like are more clearly experiential.

The contributions of phenomenological psychology and existentialism are consonant with this trend. Their emphasis on higher functioning is evident in such specific topics as the existential explorations of freedom, choice, responsibility, and meaning; and the phenomenological studies of human action, forms of spatiality, and "lived moment" by Straus (1966). An experiential focus is seen also in phenomenology's insistence on taking man as an experiencing being, and on studying the essential structures as well as the variant modes of his experience. Implicit in this particular grounding of psychology in experience is the further notion that the study of human psychology is properly the study of a "special type of order" (Gendlin, 1962, p. 21). Within this trend is the central concern with the image of man which psychology projects as a science of man.

This concern is illustrated by the so-called Third Wave, or Humanistic Psychology. As its name suggests this movement urges an orientation which would redress what is felt to be an undue stress in psychology on the mechanistic, the fragmented, and the animal (Severin, 1965, pp. xiv-xvii). The general effort is to deal with themes and phenomena which accentuate man's essential uniqueness from other life and machines. An intended by-product of this effort is an elevation of the view of man and of one of the fields of his study, psychology. One specific corrective often proffered in this movement and elsewhere is a shift from consideration of man as object to man as subject.* For phenomenology defines man as just

*Two major works which treat the image of man projected by the social sciences and psychology and which are sympathetic to this particular corrective are Matson's *Broken Image* (1964) and Koestler's *The Ghost in the Machine* (1967).

this, a subject, that is, an experiencing being. Another modification to which phenomenological psychology and existentialism can contribute is in changing the unit of study in psychology. Units which underscore the integrity of the person are available. Mode of being, mode of relatedness, and posture to the world can complement stimulus and response, drive and introjection, and trait and role.

Changing the philosophy of science

There has been a trend toward modifying the philosophy of science underlying psychology. In particular, the "caution-inspired epistemology" (Koch in Wann, 1964, p. 22) of logical positivism is being infused with a logic of inquiry based on a more personal view of knowledge. It is a view of knowledge more embedded in "the world as directly experienced" (Merleau-Ponty, 1962, viii). The shift is also from a philosophy of science which presumes and requires a full prior formulation of the logic of inquiry to one which "acknowledges the dependency of theory construction and use at every phase on individual sensitivity, discrimination, insight, judgement, guess" (Koch in Wann, 1964, pp. 21–22). With this shift there is no need to favor the selection of phenomena which are more readily observed, operationalized, and manipulated.

Polanyi, who gives this emerging philosophy of science one of its most comprehensive and popular statements, writes:

Upon examining the grounds on which science is pursued, I found that it is determined at every stage by undefinable powers of thought. No rule can account for the ways a good idea is produced for starting an enquiry; and there are no rules either for the verification or the refutation of a proposed solution of a problem. [1964, p. ix]

Polanyi describes a structure of knowledge or of knowing in which tacit knowing is more fundamental than explicit knowing. There is a knowing which is before and sometimes beyond our "telling" of it, and which we know by "dwelling" in it. Maslow, in like manner, distinguishes between spectator knowing and experiential knowing (1966, pp. 45–66). Phenomenology, analogously but more radically, builds its philosophy on the priority and primacy of experience both as the foundation of knowledge and the vehicle of knowing:

To return to things themselves as experienced is to return to that world which precedes knowledge, of which knowledge always *speaks,* and in relation to which every scientific schematization is an abstract derivative sign language. . . . [Merleau-Ponty, 1962, p. ix]

These ideas on the personal and experiential basis of knowledge question the traditional positivistic notion of objectivity. The inseparability of knowledge and our experience of it precludes the ideal of an objective stance, the notion that the observer can occupy a position or vantage point external to the object of his investigation. A somewhat different but related critique of traditional objectivism has arisen also in modern physics. It is based on the discovery that for some phenomena our measuring rod necessarily intrudes itself into the measure to a degree that the phenomena must remain always in some respects indeterminate. Again, we cannot fully "see" the object from a position external to it. We must approach the phenomenon to "have" it; and our approach to it is inseparable from our having of it.

Ironically, the realization that all knowledge is originally personal or experiential in nature allows and buttresses the kind of enlargement, described above, of the subject matter in the field of psychology. If in intelligent inquiry, as this emerging philosophy of science informs us, there is never an external "objective" observer, then inquiry into those more personal, more private, subjective, and experiential realms does not have to attempt (since it is now held impossible) to remain in a position external to them. We no longer have to favor selection of phenomena which are more readily made visible, public, "objective," and which are more readily operationalized, quantified, and the like. We can recognize openly what has always been true, that, particularly in a human science, the observer is also the object of observation.

The contribution of psychotherapy

Developments in psychotherapy parallel and complement the first two threads. We refer particularly to the following: the contribution of Rogers and its refinement by Gendlin, the whole sensitivity training and encounter movement, Perls's Existential Gestalt therapy, and the influence of phenomenological psychology and existential analysis on psychotherapy (see May et al., *Existence*, 1958; Van den Berg, *The Phenomenological Approach to Psychiatry*, 1955; and Sonneman, *Existence and Psychotherapy*, 1954). These therapies and therapists in common deemphasize genetics, causality, taxonomy, understanding by objectification, and analysis of a "psyche" conceived of as an encrusted structure. There is, instead, an emphasis on present experiencing, on increased sensitivity to one's self as an experiencing being, and on personal growth. To understand this presently existing experiencing person in these therapies is to know the world-for-him. To reach him and to help him are to "enter into" his world (Van den Berg), or to teach him to "focus" in on it (Gendlin), or to facilitate his inhabiting its opposing parts (Perls), or to have an encounter with him (May).

Newly acceptable modes of inquiry

A fourth thread involves research methods, the question of how to proceed in investigating a psychological problem. With it we return more directly to a central purpose of the present work, the application of experiential approaches and their use in conjunction with empirical methods. In a way the trends here are least clear. There has been a plethora of statements which are not much more than negative pronouncements against one or another aspect of the positivistic status quo.

In fact, though, there has been a general broadening by some investigators in modes of inquiry. This is seen, for example, in a loosening of the definition of what is acceptable as evidence. In traditional inquiry assertion is restricted to data where data are a set of quantitatively expressed results derived from the manipulation of operationalized variables in a controlled setting. A rigid application of this definition of evidence has given way in some quarters, with, of course, a backlash effect in others. A second example is the increased use of the natural setting, notably in European ethology and more recently in social psychology. The idea that inquiry may take a number of different forms and that form may be dictated in large part by the phenomena studied is being superimposed on traditional methodology. Some of this is simply the perennial tug-of-war in psychology between the legitimate advantages gained by tight controls in research, so we "will know what we have," and the strait-jacketing effects these constraints can have when too strictly applied on the freedom to explore new and interesting directions.

But, it seems to us, there are at least the makings here of a more stable shift, an alteration in the character of the mode of inquiry in the field. One of its centers, if not the center, is the experiential point of view: the study of phenomena as experienced. This vantage point is not entirely new in psychology. In 1949, Snygg and Combs presented what they referred to as a "phenomenological" psychology. However, even with this work and with the work of Lewin, Murray, and others, until quite recently the potential impact of the experiential point of view on the question of how to proceed has remained latent. While a number of reasons for this are apparent, such as the toughmindedness of the American character, establishmentarianism, or, as we mentioned earlier, the adulation of the ways of physics, an additional reason now emerges, namely, the lack of a philosophy of science comparable to and competitive with logical positivism.

It is the premise of the present work that phenomenology will provide the necessary alternative. In fact, in phenomenology, chiefly in the writings of Husserl and Merleau-Ponty but also of Sartre and Heidegger and in the psychology of Straus, Van den Berg, Van Kaam, Gendlin and others, the trends we have exposed are integrated and comprehensively treated. First, there is an acceptance of any phenomenon that has an appearance in experience, no matter how dim or transient or "unreal" that appearance might be. Second, the inclusion of any fact that constitutes "world" for a person contributes the elements of respect called for in a humanistic approach. Third, it is a philosophy of science whose epistemology is built on the fact of man's inherence or embeddedness in the world. This philosophy demonstrates the origin of knowledge in a lived or prereflective experience. It constructs a notion of "verification" based not on an idealization of the object, on the one hand, or on an isolated reflectivity by the observer on the other; but on the immediate givenness of experience and on the problem of intersubjectivity. Fourth, phenomenonology includes a carefully worked out posture to the other and to his world which has already provided the basis for a description of psychopathology (Van den Berg, 1955; Straus, 1966; Binswanger, in May et al., 1958) and for various therapies (Gendlin, 1969; Perls, 1969; Boss, 1963).

Part of our advocacy of phenomenology is based on the belief that it can contribute to an emerging identity for psychology, an identity which establishes it as a field between the natural sciences and the humanities, as a peculiarly human science.

Having spelled out these general views, we return to the more specific context of the methodological approach we shall take. While there are by now in the literature analyses of various problems employing a phenomenological method, there are few attempts to integrate this approach with empirical or experimental methods. For example, most of the articles in the recently founded *Journal of Phenomenological Psychology* are purely descriptive, nonempirical efforts. In most investigations that do put the phenomenological and the experimental together only a propaedeutic role is given to the former. (MacLeod, in Wann, 1964, explicitly limits phenomenology's role to this.) A phenomenological method is used as an aid in generating ideas or in clarifying the phenomenon prior to the study proper. It is a kind of procedure to formalize the productive engagement which occurs while the investigator is shaving or showering, before he actually arrives at the laboratory.

Another only marginal or peripheral use of the experiential in research method is exemplified by Rogers's work in psychotherapy. In this research most of the variables are experiential ("positive regard," empathy and the like) while the methodology is traditional (Hart and Tomlinson, 1970). Measures of the target variables consist of various scales and observer or even participant ratings. Goals are correlations among the variables and predicted outcomes, usually of therapeutic change or success. The subject matter is centrally experiential but the investigatory stance is objectivist. We "see" and work with positive regard, for example, from outside of the thing itself.

An additional stage, this time at least in the direction of a more genuine or truly integrative method, is exemplified by the Van Kaam study mentioned earlier (1966). Here again, the target phenomenon is explicitly experiential, the experience of "being really understood." But the goal now is a description of the phenomenon as experienced. It is no longer to construct, through successful predictions, a network of relations among phenomena. However, the method, as distinguished from the goal of the investigation, is still essentially objectivistic. The investigator asks a group of subjects to describe the target phenomenon by recourse to their own experience. He then analyzes the resultant protocols by objectively abstracting their common elements. The investigator remains or attempts to remain at all times outside the phenomenon. He at no point himself assumes an experiential stance to the phenomenon.

The general approach of this paper takes very seriously the experiential point of view. It attempts to employ it as an investigatory stance and as a way to proceed which may be integrated with controlled data gathering and experimental hypothesis testing, as well as with clinically derived and intuitively derived theory. We shall describe the stance more fully in the third chapter immediately prior to the descriptive formulation of introversion. The stance relies heavily on a modification of Gendlin's notion of the interaction between felt-meaning and reflected thought, between experience as bodily felt and our conceptualization of it. Also in that section, we shall review some of the substantive results of phenomenology. These are constitutive features of experience which will provide a general descriptive form for our particular problem, a phenomenological description of introversion.

The plan of the work more specifically is first to consider a clinically derived theory and to explicate it. Jung's theory of introversion is both the seminal work and, even to the present, the most well developed theory in the literature. Our assumption here is that however objectified and reductive the language employed, the theories of giant thinkers, like Freud, Jung, and others, contain an experiential bedrock. This bedrock, once explicated, can be utilized by adopting an experiential point of view to it.

A second step, preparatory to the experiential formulation, is to gather data with standard empirical procedures. We shall present an investigation involving a projective technique, the Thematic Apperception Test. We initially worked with this material much as had Van Kaam. We abstracted elements which distinguish the protocols of those subjects labelled introverts from those labelled extraverts.

Finally we shall assume an experiential stance to both sets of guidelines, the theoretical and the empirical, to reconcile them with the phenomenon as experienced. This particular use of phenomenological procedure as an investigatory stance and a descriptive framework has some claim to originality. To the degree that it is successful, it may align traditional objective methods with emerging phenomenological ones, moving toward a more integrative approach to problems in personality.

1. The Theoretical Referent: The Jungian Concept

The Problem of Introversion

Is there anything there?

Since Jung first popularized the term "introversion" with the publication of *Psychological Types* in 1923, the literature of personality has been permeated with studies on introversion and introversion-extraversion (I/E) related variables. A glance at the bibliography of two review articles will verify this assertion (Carrigan, 1960; Dicks-Mireaux, 1964). In addition, there are a large number of personality variables which could be properly considered derivatives of I/E and which have enjoyed widespread attention, such as inner- and outer-directedness, field dependence and field independence, etc. The practice of employing moderator variables, prevalent in much current personality research (Wallach, 1967), offers still another demonstration of the pervasiveness of the I/E variable, and, presumably, of its felt-importance and centrality. While we have made no actual count, it is clear that one or another measure of I/E is among the most frequently used moderators, along with gender and some measure of neuroticisms or adjustment. And yet despite this, or because of this proliferating influence, one of the conclusions of the Carrigan review article mentioned above is that "curiously, there is little agreement as to the meaning of I/E" (1960, p. 330). Consensus is lacking both as to the concept and its referent.

More surprising still than this conceptual disparity among measures of I/E, but perhaps related to it, is the paucity of attempts to work out the concept in any detail. There have been at least two attempts to abstract and analyze the descriptive as distinguished from the theoretical statements in Jung's writings on the types (Guilford, 1940; Cook, 1970). But there is, at least to our knowledge, no formal attempt in the literature to pull together Jung's theoretical statements about I/E. As we will describe, in the place of a carefully worked out formulation there are numerous sets of unidimensional polarities, unintegrated and at variance with one another even within a set. When we turn to a different literature, one somewhat outside of academic psychology, the several expositors who have written the basic "primers" of Jungian psychology, typically practicing Jungian clinicians, devote only limited discussion to introversion itself or to the I/E distinction (see for examples: Fordham, 1956; Jacobi, 1962; and Bennett, 1967). Of these Bennett offers the most detailed discussion and also the one which is most congruent with the formulation developed in the present paper (pp. 50–54). But these writers, including Bennett, focus more on the working of the typology as a whole, on the relation of I/E to the functions,* and on the principle of opposites (defined and discussed below) than on introversion or the I/E distinction per se.

Jung's writings on I/E in comparison are lengthy and comprehensive. He chooses to give a pivotal role to this distinction in his general theory of personality. His *Psychological Types* is a 600-page treatise devoted to a thorough exposition of the terms introversion and extraversion. Jung accomplishes this exposition by examining variant expressions of the I/E difference through history, in philosophical, literary, and scholarly writings; I/E in combination with the psychological functions; I/E in different cultural contexts; and I/E conceptualized, as we will see, in more than one theoretical framework.

How, then, do we understand this disjunction between Jung's relatively full-bodied concept of introversion and its simplification into a number of discrepant and disjointed polarities? One interpretation of the situation asserts that assuming the integrity of introversion as a phenomenon was unwarranted, that Jung's "introvert" does not exist in nature. In this view, Jung rightfully is credited with the contribution of a broad-ranging and pioneering work which itself located various individual differences in personality and pointed the way to numerous others. However, this view goes on, the umbrella under which Jung placed these variable aspects was leaky from the outset. Jung simply erred in integrating some elements that do not necessarily occur together. There is no basic type, no genotype, introversion. What we have called the proliferation of I/E-related variables is, more accurately, the separation of more or less unrelated and distinct aspects of personality. There are various I/E measures,

---

*In Jung's typology, in addition to the two attitudes I/E, there are four basic psychological functions: Thinking, feeling, sensation, and intuition. There are, then, four main introverted types and four extraverted types, although the typology eventually differentiates further beyond these eight through the consideration of a second or "auxiliary" function.

various "related" dimensions, and various moderators because there exist these phenomena which are discrete and for which there need be no overarching concept, no integrative theory. Introversion, to conclude this view, is a fruitful progenitor but one which died in childbirth.

Although these conclusions are plausibly derived from a reading of the literature in this area of personality, they are implausible in the face of the existence of the phenomenon. Outside of psychology do we not use the terms "introversion" and "extraversion"? Has not the culture readily "found" the two types, and, as it were, populated itself with them? We all know, for example, the introvert, that somewhat opaque, asocial, and aloof individual, that museum-goer, or mathematician, or "loner" in whatever walk of life. We know immediately that there is something about him that is not the pathological isolation of the schizoid or the alienated individual; and with as much certainty we perceive about him a same something that distinguishes him from the extravert. We recognize immediately, without reflection, introvertedness. We know its appearance. But we want to know how to understand it, how to say what it is; and we want to know what it is to live it.

Even within the field, among psychologists who are interested in this area of personality, undoubtedly among also the very psychologists whose reading of the literature finds no unified or unifiable notion of introversion, the term "introvert" is still a meaningful one. In fact, a disproportionate number of psychologists consider themselves, and if given the opportunity will describe themselves, as introverts. Introvertedness points to a specific though complex something for them, to some distinct aspects or qualities of their personality. That this is the case was confirmed for us in the context of some weekly meetings several years ago of psychologists interested in the Jungian typology. These meetings established that the group shared some common views on the Jungian attitudes I/E. There was striking agreement on which of several individuals known to all were introverts (I's) and which were extraverts (E's). There was also considerable agreement in labeling particular traits and behaviors that entered the discussion as introverted or extraverted. The meetings also reconfirmed, however, the difficulty in making explicit a concept of introversion. While there were intuitive nods around the table, it was an instance of "knowing more than we can tell" (Polanyi, 1966, p.4).

Such a situation breeds both excitement and frustration. In this case it raised in relief the problem of the present paper, how to proceed in the study of personality. How are we to locate and formulate these shared and pervasive but seemingly ineffable aspects of personality?

Our starting point, at any rate, is that the integrity of the phenomenon is a consensually verifiable and verified fact. There are one or more identifiable aspects of personality which are what is introverted about an introvert. The disagreement, as Carrigan noted, is in the meaning and the formulation of introversion (1960). The problem is how to arrive at saying what it is and what kinds of terms to employ for this task.

The literature since Jung

What is Jung's concept of introversion; and why, given his presentation of it, is there still disagreement about the meaning of it? What questions does he leave unanswered? How did he proceed to unearth a powerful aspect of personality and somehow simultaneously to lay the groundwork for its present conceptual muddiness? Before we address these questions through an exposition of Jung's writings on introversion, let us briefly review the development of these concepts since Jung. This will highlight further the "problem" of introversion and the appropriateness of the methodology we will be applying to the problem in the present work.

Stanfiel (1964) gives a brief history of work on I/E in this country from its inception in the 1920s. Through the twenties and thirties the primary concern was to develop psychometrically rigorous instruments with which to measure I/E. As Stanfiel suggests (p. 95), to incorporate certain desirable psychometric properties into their instruments, investigators felt compelled to modify the Jungian concept. In particular, they simplified it.

Later, several inventories appeared purporting to measure I/E (specifically, for example, Myers-Briggs, 1962; Gray-Wheelwright, 1946). At this point several investigators attempted to bring these inventories together and analyze them through the technique of factor analysis. This was in the interest of a kind of purification, an effort to distill from them those aspects occurring in common. These factors might then be held to constitute the I/E difference. Guilford's earlier work (1930, 1940) was seminal. He extracted factors from the various inventories as well as from Jung's descriptions of the introverted and extraverted types. At one point he obtained five factors. Defining them in the introverted direction, these were: social introversion, a tendency to be disaffiliative; thinking introversion, an inclination to be introspective, meditative; depression, a pessimistic outlook as distinguished from an optimistic, outgoing disposition; cycloid disposition, emotional stability for the *I*; and rathymia, inhibition, overcontrol of impulses. Among factors associated with I/E by other workers particularly Cattell (Carrigan, 1960), are included: general activity, less tendency for action in the *I;* autia, emphasis on subjectivity and inner mental life; and dominance, less in the *I.*

It is clear that the factor analytic studies of Guilford, Cattell, Eysenck, and others, even taken singly, increased the divergence of conceptions of introversion and extraversion. We have only hinted at the serpentine movement of these developments. A retrospective view suggests an unending exercise in both factor analytic method and the construction of psychometric instruments. For example, Guilford initially obtained four factors from the various extant inventories. From these he devised his own inventory (Guilford, 1940) and factor analyzed it, yielding the five factors we listed above. These were later incorporated into a new inventory which in turn was factor analyzed by North, yielding two factors (Stanfiel, 1964, p. 101).

There is little attempt on the part of these investigators to integrate factors into a coherent and cogent definition of introversion or extraversion.* Rather, as we mentioned, they began to speak of kinds of introversion and kinds of extraversion (Stanfiel, 1964, p. 102). Murray, following a different path, also arrived at the conclusion that one needs to define different types of introversion and extraversion (1938, p. 242). Carrigan (1960), reviewing work since 1953, concluded that I/E is a demonstrably pervasive aspect of personality, but that it has not been demonstrated to be a unitary dimension of personality.

The divergence of notions of I/E and the disparity among them is, then, a main product of the work of this period. The conception of the phenomenon which Jung initially described was dispersed and

---

*Eysenck is an exception here in that he eventually elaborated an integrated concept of "extraversion." He, however, disclaims that his concept has any source in or relation to the thinking of Jung (Eysenck, 1967). His concept centers on a "constitutional" or physiological individual difference in degree of cortical inhibition and explicitly builds on the writings of Pavlov, Hull, Kohler, and Klein and Krech (Eysenck, 1955).

in disarray. But it was at the same time, as Stanfiel notes, simplified conceptually. For underlying the catalogue of unintegrated factors or polarities of this period and the later derivatives of them in the personality literature, there is a simplistic conceptual framework. It derives from a superficial reading of Jung on I/E. As we shall describe, Jung grappled with the problem of the role of the subject and the object in perception and in experience. His distinction between I/E is built on this problem. It is a complex and enigmatic one philosophically, as well as psychologically. Jung's insight is that these two possible facets or sides of perception or experience provide the basis for a fundamental difference in personality among people. An individual consistently, but not exclusively, orients himself toward one or the other of these aspects, either toward the subject or the object. The conceptual framework, or loose organizing principle, originates in a translation of Jung's various and peculiar usages of "subject" and "subjective" into "inside" and, similarly, "object" and "objective" into "outside."

The pervasive polarity in/out or inside/outside, where "in" is associated with introversion and "out" with extraversion, influences all notions of I/E in the literature since Jung. With this starting point the variables we are reviewing then center on an answer to one of two questions about introversion: What is it that is inside (the filler question); and of what is it composed (the container question)? The various unintegrated answers to these questions constitute the conceptual literature of I/E since Jung and some main threads of more recent derivative personality research. To illustrate, inside/outside have been taken variously as mental/physical, which has in turn been rendered as ideas/things, thinking/acting, and ideas/facts; self/others; inhibition/impulsivity; internal mediation/external reactivity; body/field; internal standards/external standards; passivity/activity; internal/external locus of control; internal/external locus of attention.* In each instance the first involves either an internal filler or a container. For example, inhibition is keeping feelings and/or actions inside, while body is a container.

It is obvious from this listing that an inside/outside distinction as

*Ideas/facts has been emphasized by the Myers-Briggs Test Inventory (Myers, 1962); self/others has been emphasized in factor analytic work and in the Myers-Briggs; inhibition/impulsivity by Guilford and Eysenck. Internal mediation/external reactivity has been studied by Kagan (1966; "reflectivity/impulsivity"); body/field by Witkin et al. (1962; "field independence/dependence"); internal/external standards by Riesman (1963; "inner/outer directed"); internal/external locus of control by Rotter (Gore and Rotter, 1963); internal/external locus of attention by J. Singer (1966).

a basis of individual differences is a productive one. The translation of Jung's subjective/objective into inside/outside has generated other personality variables which themselves have been useful tools for the understanding of individual differences. The search for fillers and containers has been productive and undoubtedly will yield additional variables, but it has not captured Jung's original insight about I/E. It fails to mirror faithfully Jung's concept both by oversimplifying it and by fractionating it without putting it back together again. The translation has not been productive if our goal is to understand what Jung means and what we, in everyday usage, mean by introversion and extraversion.

For example, Jung is not saying that an *I* is an idea person or thinking person while an *E* is a factual or acting person. Clearly everyone lives in a world of both ideas and facts, of both thought and action. Such distinctions may account for some of the variance in a sample of *I*s and *E*s. A hypothesis based on these or other polarities may yield statistically significant results, although we believe that to attain such results one must either limit the polarity to a very particular situation or moderate it with a second variable (see Shapiro and Alexander, 1969). But this framework, which is productive in its own right, has not captured or clarified Jung's concept of I/E. It has lost it, as we have indicated by pointing to the disagreement about the meaning of I/E and the disparity among measures, "factors," and operations of it. We have argued that what has been lost is not only a theory or concept but also a phenomenon of personality which we all recognize and employ in daily life.

To study the phenomenon of introversion we must first recognize what kind of "thing" it is. Only then can we fashion the method to approach it, the kind of concepts to capture it, and the appropriate terms to describe it. Jung's theory tells us that the I/E distinction is an attitudinal difference. By "attitude" Jung refers to a stance toward or a particular view of the world, of one's self in it, and of one's mental processes or experiencing. An attitude in this sense is a subtle, postural phenomenon, one that generally is only tacitly felt by the attitude holder and yet is undeniably present for him in all situations; and one which may only be erratically manifest to others in any particular action of its holder and yet that in large part constitutes for others his "personality," his particularity. Because it is an attitudinal phenomenon, introversion cannot be studied exclusively through an operation of it. We cannot deal exclusively in attempts to objectify it, to see it as an object or as it appears to others in action or gesture. The central task in the problem of introversion is to describe a particular view of the world, as it is viewed, and to find concepts that capture a particular way of being in the world.

To accomplish this, we require a method which allows us to hold onto this particular attitude, to continually approach the phenomenon in experience. We require a method which is an ongoing arbitration between the phenomenon as it is given in experience and objectivist, empirical data. In this way the phenomenon can remain focal and full-bodied. While we may temporarily simplify it, reduce it, or fractionate it, since we maintain access to it we prevent our own methodological nets from strangling it. Our operation of it or our inventory or measure of it, does not become the phenomenon itself.

Again, we shall describe this integrated method in chapter 3. Here we want only to indicate how the need for such a method grows out of the nature of understanding introversion as well as out of the history and manner of its study.

Definitions

We begin the exposition of Jung on introversion with two definitions given in *Psychological Types.* The labels heading the two definitions will become clear in a moment. In chapter 10 of that book, which is the main expositional chapter on the typology, Jung defines introversion as follows:

First definition—the Structural Model

The introvert interposes a subjective view between the perception of the object and his own action, which prevents the action from assuming a character that corresponds with the objective situation. [p. 471]

In the glossary to *Psychological Types,* an extensive chapter which deals with all the major concepts and terms of the theory, he makes the following definitive statement:

Second definition—the Energy Model

Introversion means a turning inward of the libido, whereby a negative relation of subject to object is expressed. Interest does not move towards the object but recedes towards the subject. [p. 567]

Finally, as a working reference, we shall quote an example of the I/E distinction, one which Jung employs at the beginning of chapter 10.

Because it is cold out of doors, one man [the *E*] is persuaded to wear his overcoat, another [the *I*] from a desire to become hardened finds this unnecessary. [p. 416]

As one reads the two definitions of introversion, while it is not altogether clear what they are saying, it is clear that each is saying something somewhat different. One points to the "interposition of a subjective view"; the other refers to "an inward turning of the libido." It is a central thesis of our exposition of Jung on introversion that the two definitions may be understood in terms of two models of introversion found in *Psychological Types.* The two models are implicit in that they are not labeled as constructs by Jung and in that they are not explicitly distinguished from each other. Not only does each model provide a definition of introversion, each provides its own language, the terms of which pervade much of Jung's material on introversion. We should note also that none of the several foremost disciples and expositors of Jung mentioned earlier makes explicit either the two models or the two ways in which Jung apparently thought about introversion. A main task of this chapter will be to explicate these two models.

Paralleling Freud's general theory of mind, Jung's first complete theory of mind, which has as its center the theoretical constructs introversion-extraversion, consists of a structural model and a dynamic model. A structural model generally presents a topography or map of mind; while a dynamic model ideally describes the modes or principles of transport from one region to another on the map. It is perhaps a sign of Jung's genius that he, like Freud, proceeded with more than one model at once. But as we try to arrive at the phenomenon he called introversion, at his understanding of this phenomenon, and at the experience that is peculiarly introverted, this sign of Jung's intellectual stature only increases our task.

Structural Model

Background of the I/E distinction: The problem of the role of the subject and object in perception

One of the fundamental problems in the history of philosophy is that of the relation between reality and our knowledge of it; it is the question What is? and the inseparable question How do we know what is? It is the question of the relation between what is out there and what we perceive: Of that which we perceive, what is in the perceiver, the subject, and what is in the perceived, the object? Is what we perceive what is, or do we create it in our perception? These are ontological and epistemological concerns of philosophy.

Jung was quite aware of these problems and of philosophy's treatment of them. Several sections of *Psychological Types* review the history of philosophy of classical and medieval times. We mention Jung's sophistication and learning in this area because his insight about introversion and extraversion has such questions as its context or background.

To begin to develop this context, let us compare Jung to other psychologists in their approaches to an issue related to these questions. Psychologists, of course, are interested in the determinants of perception or consciousness. A psychological rendering of the philosophical problems above is as follows: What are the roles of the subject and the object in what we perceive? What is the role of the perceiver, the subject, in what we perceive; and what is the role of the perceived, the object of our perception, in what we perceive? Most psychologists approach this problem by attempting to sort out those characteristics of the subject and those properties of the object which may be said to determine perception, or consciousness more generally. They begin with the observation that people vary in their perception of what is apparently the same situation. They ask what is it about people and what is it about objects or situations that determine this variance.

In thinking about the subjective determinants, for example, an investigator might examine an individual's perceptual apparatus, or his history of perceptions, or his present "need-states." Objective determinants might involve various physical, contextual, or aspectival properties of the object of consciousness. An investigator would by proceeding in this way arrive at a statement as to how in general these factors contribute to a person's consciousness at any given moment and how they explain or account for the observed individual variance in perception or consciousness.

Jung approaches the problem of the determinants of consciousness and of the role of the subjective and objective factors in this determination in his own peculiar way. His starting point is not the common observation of the variability of perception from individual to individual, although in his general theory of personality he does account eventually for this variance. He begins, rather, with an observation such as the one in the example earlier of the cold weather. His observation is that there are two classes of people. They differ in that they process the same information or situation (the weather) differently. Jung's primary observation is that there are two kinds of "perceivers" in the world.

Aside from the question of its validity, how is it that Jung finds two classes of people and focuses on this discovery while most other psychologists focus on an observed fact of general variability? There is more to understanding Jung's peculiar starting point than simply to note that he has a typological approach to personality. This only moves the question back a step to how it is that he arrived at a typological approach. Further, as we have mentioned and will describe below, his theory by no means is restricted to a scheme of grouping individuals by type. It eventually presents an explanation of the general individual variance in perception and consciousness. Nor is it entirely sufficient to understand his focus on the fact of twoness, to know that thinking in two category sets was a central mode of intellectual thought of the day (Kaufmann, 1965, pp. 167–175). As we will see, particularly in his "principle of opposites," Jung's theories at almost every point proceed by two.

Jung is struck by the fact of twoness because of his familiarity with the philosophical issues we described. He becomes aware that there are two classes of perceivers because he has examined the history of philosophy and noted a repeated opposition between different schools at various periods. There is always one school which dwells on the subject, the person, as the center of reality or the ground of knowledge. This is, for example, the idealist's position. There is always a second school which emphasizes the concrete existence of the object of perception, the world, as the prior reality, the realist's position. At any given time in the history of philosophy Jung observes that there are these two strains of thought which differ in that they focus on one of the two possible fulcrums to explain consciousness and the world—the perceiver or the perceived, the knower or the known, the subject or the object.

In fact, as Bennett points out, Jung in his *Two Essays on Analytical Psychology* viewed the relatively short history of psychology in similar terms (1967). For Jung, the psychologies of Freud and Adler illustrate an analogous difference. He sees in them " 'a contrast between two different types of human mentality, one of which finds the determining agency pre-eminently in the subject, the other in the object' " (1967, p. 50).

Jung does not choose to focus on the problem of individual variance, although he is well aware of its existence. He does not try to locate the various subjective and objective determinants of consciousness. Instead, he is attuned to the fact that there are these two necessary bases of perception and of consciousness, the perceiver or subject and the perceived or object. So primed, he "discovers" the two personality classes which he terms introversion and extraversion. Upon this distinction he builds his first theory of personality.

In a way, with his I/E distinction, what Jung has done with respect to some fundamental problems in philosophy and psychology is facile; and, in a way, it is elegant. From one point of view, he has begged the philosophical question or dilemma of what is the proper and original grounding of reality, the knower or the known, world-creator or world. He has also begged the psychological question as to the sorting out of the respective roles of the subjective and of the objective in an individual's consciousness. His "answer" is the clear equivocation: There are two classes of individuals, the one oriented to the subject in consciousness, the other to the object.

But from another point of view what Jung has perpetrated is a dazzling coup in the history of ideas. He has taken the two horns of a fundamental dilemma and hung on each an orientation which power-fully defines one of the two classes of people. In an equally dazzling stroke he uses his insight about I/E to psychologize away the various schools of philosophy which have attempted to deal with the dilem-ma. He attributes their respective philosophical positions to the personalitics of their respective proponents. There generally have been two schools of philosophy differing along the lines we have described because there are two basic personality types. Idealism, for example, is a reflection of the attitude of an *I*, while realism is a manifestation of an *E*'s orientation.

With this background a generic definition of I/E, one which encompasses the two definitions which we quoted at the outset, may be stated: An *I* is a member of a class of individuals who are oriented predominantly to the subject as the basis of their consciousness, while an *E* is a member of a class of individuals oriented more to the object as the basis of their consciousness. The structural and dynamic models of I/E will present two "explanations" of this differential orientation. They will conceptualize consciousness in terms of these two entities, the subject and the object, in ways which allow the two to be differentially dominant or determinant for the two classes of individuals. Incidentally, with this same background the problem of the experience of introversion is delimited grossly. A description of the experience of introversion requires a phenomenology of subjectivity.

Two psychic domains: The internalization of the subject and object

From his starting point, Jung then posits that the reason the *I* and the *E* have different perceptions of the same thing is that the "determinants" of their perception or consciousness are different. The determinants are two domains in the psyche. Each individual has both domains, but one or the other is "relatively more determinant" for each individual. These two domains, which are variably dominant from individual to individual, are the basis of the structural model of I/E. In this model the distinction I/E refers to a relative predominance in the feeding into consciousness of material from one or the other of these two domains.

And what are the two domains? Of course, they are derivatives of the two necessary entities in perception, the subject and the object. Jung has internalized the two entities as two psychic domains. The subject, person, or the "subjective factor," or in the first definition, that one associated with the structural model, the "subjective view," is housed in one part of the psyche, while the object or external world is housed in the second part. There exist in the psyche two domains, one of which is the subjective factor and one of which is the objective factor, and both of which have the property of feeding into or determining consciousness.

The internalization of these two traditional aspects of perception is only the first step in Jung's treatment of them in the present model. Not only are they two possible orientations toward or views of the objects constituting consciousness, they are two realities each of which provides its own orientation or view. As we noted, historically different philosophies (and psychologies) have argued that either the subject or the object is the basis of what is and/or what we know and that one or the other is the ground of reality. For Jung, they are both right. There are two realities.

Both realities are psychological, both are aspects of mind.* They are there as such, as realities given in and constituting consciousness, in each individual. Mind has this structure. Accordingly, in the structural model, each individual has available to him in consciousness, although not necessarily subject to his will, two images or facts, or ideas, or feelings. He has available two images of God, two ideas and sets of feelings of mother, and so forth, each housed in its own domain or region of mind. The two images are more or less independent of each other. Each is a reality, a constituting stuff of consciousness. Individuals differ in having one or the other of these two realities dominant.

Of one of these realities, that associated with introversion, Jung poetically tells us: "The subjective factor is something that is just as much a fact as the extent of the sea and the radius of the earth" (1923, p. 474). It is this first reality that Jung felt people did not realize and to which they needed to be introduced. This is consistent with his view that western European culture was predominantly an extraverted culture. Jung calls the psychic domain which houses this potential reality the "collective unconscious." In the first definition with which we began above, the term "subjective view" has this specific referent. That part of the "self," Jung's term for the totality of the psyche, which "interposes the subjective view is the collective unconscious" (p. 476). It is the relatively dominant determinant of the consciousness of the *I*.

The collective unconscious is a domain, a part of the psyche, in which are housed all those "psychic contents" which are "peculiar not to one individual but to many" (p. 530). It is the "symbolic transformation" of the common, the collective, or the universal. The image from this domain, for example the image of mother, need bear no relation in its particulars to the individual's actual historic mother. The contents from the domain collective unconscious "are represented in consciousness in the forms of pronounced tendencies, or definite ways of looking at things" (p. 476). For the *I*, "these

---

*That the two realities are conceived as primarily psychological realities, prior to any antecedents they might have in a present or historical external reality, makes Jung's theory of mind itself an idealistic or subjectivist theory. This characterization of Jung's theory is drawn also by Van Kaam (1966, p. 209). We shall return to this point in a later section. Here we shall note only that it is somewhat ironic in the light of our earlier discussion. Jung's theory of mind, while it takes off from the observation that historically there have been two kinds of theories of philosophy and psychology, the subjectivistic and the objectivistic, itself falls more or less exclusively into one of these camps.

subjective tendencies and ideas are stronger. . . . They are superim-posed upon all impressions" (p. 476). The subjective view, or the subjective factor in consciousness, is an increment to the objective data of perception in the form of a feed-in from the collective unconscious. This feed-in from the collective unconscious is the specific and precise construct of introversion in the structural model. The view, or as Jung on occasion more broadly describes it, the reality given by this feed-in, is the introverted attitude. We shall say more about the meaning of the linkage in this model of introversion and the collective unconscious below.

The second reality is the objective factor or view. It is the counterpart of the subjective view. Like the subjective view, it is depicted in this model by a domain of the psyche. It contains, like the subjective domain, all manner of psychic contents—facts, images, ideas, and feelings. Jung dwells on this domain much less than on the collective unconscious. He conceives of it as more closely and di-rectly related to the actual present external situation, object, or world than is the subjective domain, although its precise relation to the external world is not specified. It is, however, clearly a psychic stuff. It is not the physical world itself. What we have from Jung is that this second reality represents, in a more immediate and direct way than does the reality given by the subjective domain, the external world. The image, ideas, feelings, and the like, of mother, for example, in this domain derive in some more direct way from the individual's real mother in the flesh. The more direct representation of or derivation from the real historical mother is described by Jung in this model, and in the earlier definition associated with it, by the notion of correspondence. The image of mother given by this domain corresponds more with the actual historical mother. This domain is the predominant determinant of consciousness for the E. It is the feed-in analogous to that from the collective unconscious for the I. The view or reality so given is the extraverted attitude.

Let us turn for a moment from the structural model back to the example of the I/E distinction with which we began: It is cold outside and the I does not put a coat on while the E does. The cold is an external objective fact or situation observed in common. The I interposes a subjective view, an idea from the realm of the collective unconscious appears in consciousness. It is this view or idea that constitutes Jung's definition of introversion, not the behavior to which it leads. In this instance, the idea or view has something to do with "hardening" oneself. This idea and the consequent behavioral expression of it in some sense do not "correspond" to the objective situation. It is cold and the *I* goes without a coat.

The *E* receives in consciousness an idea which is more immediately related to the objective situation. He observes the cold and is persuaded to wear a coat to deal with this objective reality. The idea in consciousness of wearing a coat is the result of an objective view which, although it is as much an idea or feeling as is the subjective view, is somehow more directly related to the objective fact. According to the structural model, it is received from a psychic reality conceived of as a domain which is independent of the subjective domain and which provides in the psyche a view, again, somehow more immediately reflective of the actual present situation. This view and the action to which it may lead "correspond" to the objective situations.

What is meant by extraversion is really stickier than what is meant by introversion, at least in terms of this model. On the occasion of the sighting of an object, some ideas or feelings occur in consciousness. The aim of the model, as we outlined in an earlier section, is to provide two different and relatively decisive determinants of those thoughts and feelings. For one person, the *I*, some thoughts, feelings, or more broadly, ways of looking at things, are given by the collective unconscious. For a second person, an *E*, the thoughts and feelings originate in a domain the contents of which are more intimately tied to external reality, to the object. This is not to say that the *E* receives more sense data from the object than does the *I*; nor does it mean to say that the *I* has more thoughts and feelings than does the *E*. The difference is only in the respective domains from which the inner thoughts or feelings originate. For the *E*, the view supplied by the domain dominant for him is more directly representative of the occasioning situations; while the view typically given to the *I* loses some of this correspondence.

The construct of I/E obtained from the structural model is getting clearer. But the experiential question, the question of what in experience constitutes the views given by the two domains is not yet explicated.

The subjective domain: Introversion and the collective unconscious

The description of the introverted view as distinct from the extraverted may be pursued further within the terms of the structural model by examining the implications of Jung's explicit linking of introversion to the collective unconscious. In what sense does Jung mean that the view given by the latter is "subjective"?

We argued earlier that the description of introversion and extraversion solves the basic problem of the role of the subject and object in perception by internalizing and topographically locating the two roles in two discrete psychic domains. We also noted that in treating this problem other psychological theories typically offer concepts which are intended to explain or to account for the observed individual variance in perception. While both subjective and objective factors are implicated in most theories, it is the former, the subjective factors, which bear most of this burden of accounting for the "individualistic" character of perception. Popular usage of the term "subjective" supports this point. Of course, the term carries innumerable meanings and connotations, but it usually implies that which is individualistic. In conversational use, we often preface a view which we feel less assured that others will share with us, with the qualifier, "This is just my subjective impression. . . ."*

It may seem from a reading of the first definition of introversion, the one associated with the structural model, that the I, consistent with this emphasis on the subjective as the individualistic, has a more variable response or view than does the E. The I's view, after all, does not "correspond" to the actual present situation. If this is so we should expect that his response would appear to an onlooker to be more individualistic, more nonconformist, more variable. But, on closer inspection, the definition and the model do not imply that there is more variability of views from I to I than there is from E to E. That an E's response or view in some sense corresponds to the objective situation more than does that of an I does not necessarily imply this. The variability of perceptions that do not correspond with the actual present situation may be no greater than those that do if the former also have their own limiting "situation," the contents of the collective unconscious. This still leaves the logical possibility that while the views of Is are not in actual fact more variable than those of Es, because of their peculiar origin, they give that appearance to others. We shall defer discussion of this possibility for a later section where we treat the I's typical appearance to others.

*In a different context, R. D. Laing makes the same point: "It is interesting, for example, that one frequently encounters 'merely' before subjective, whereas it is almost inconceivable to speak of anyone being 'merely' objective" (1965, p. 25).

We bring up this possible misreading of the first definition of introversion, a misreading which might be reinforced by popular usage of the term "subjective" because, while both definitions point to an association of subjective with the "individualistic," with the idiosyncratic, and with greater individual variability, the term as it is employed in the structural model leads to a radically different association. It is crucial to understand what this particular meaning of subjective is, since the term is central to both the structural and the dynamic models.

In the structural model, "subjective view" has its origin in the collective unconscious. This latter construct is not an easy one to fathom but some points are clear. This is a domain whose contents (or stored potential contents) are common to at least those persons sharing a common cultural heritage. They are contents that are collective, and universal. They are anything but individualistic or idiosyncratic. In fact, Jung defines "collective" by distinguishing it from its opposite, those individualistic traits which are more superficial and which compose an individual's outer "personality" (Serrano, 1966, p. 54).

By virtue of this origin the subjective view, the relatively more dominant view of the I, is more universal or collective than that of the E. This contrast holds in the sense that the E's view is more anchored in the objective situation of the moment in its particularity. The I's view is more anchored in a form or theme of that situation which has been general or typical to situations of that kind through a historical period.

As we noted earlier, it is this subjective factor, this one of two realities, whose existence and effects Jung feels he needs to introduce and to demonstrate. He saw the culture in which he wrote as an extraverted culture, a culture where the object is dominant and not the subject. Even the Is in this culture, because of the "generally accepted extraverted view," "look without not behind their consciousness" (1923, p. 477), i.e., even the I, in whom the subjective factor is necessarily dominant, is unaware of its existence and influence.

Jung begins, as we have seen, by observing that there are two different classes of people, distinguished by attitude. One of these, the Is, are the kinds of people who do not wear a coat when it is cold outside; nor do they, to give another of Jung's examples, share the admiration of others for the new tenor (1923, p. 416). Their behavior does not correspond in some sense to the objective situation. In the popularly accepted extraverted view which Jung found in the culture in which he lived, these people are at best a bit odd, idiosyncratic, whimsical; at worst, they are egotistical, bizarre, withdrawn.

In Jung's conception, however, this class, the *I*s, are not more variable in their view or more individualistic or whimsical; they are nonconformists only from the point of view of *E*s and an extraverted culture. The *I* is governed, in this conception, by a different reality than is the *E*. We will assert that by associating him with the subjective view Jung felt he was rescuing the *I*. He was saving this person who seems to see things so oddly and whimsically from any aberrant or pathological tinge. He was recasting him and elevating him, not only to equality with his counterpart *E*, but perhaps even above him. It is the *I* who is more governed by something subjective and not by the idiosyncratic or the autistic. What Jung basically meant by subjective is what the term commonly means in philosophy, not in psychology or popular usage. While the objective refers to the external world, the subjective is that which is peculiar to the nature of man, that which most essentially constitutes the subject, man. The domain of the collective unconscious represents this for Jung and led to his fascination with it. He felt it housed in some distillate form the history of man's experience. It is, as is so graphically and literally demonstrated in the present model of introversion, the internalization of the subject, man. In that Jung's *I* is more governed by the rule of this domain, though neither the *I* nor those who surround him are necessarily aware of its control, he is elevated.

One further result of the linking of introversion with the collective unconscious and of the structural model in general is that the linkage dictated, in part, the subsequent direction of Jung's thinking and work. Following *Psychological Types,* Jung devoted much of his adult life to exploring and mapping out what he felt were the contents of the collective unconscious until this domain became as complex and rich as Dante's labyrinths. But with this, the task of describing what it is like to be an *I*, a task only begun in *Psychological Types,* was largely abandoned. Apparently the cost of his search for the denizens of the collective unconscious was his loss of interest in I/E itself. As we will see, by 1935 Jung presented, in a set of summary lectures, a new structural scheme of the psyche which does not even include I/E by name.

The structural model: Summary

The thorny problem of the nature of consciousness, historically addressed primarily by philosophy, provides the background or context for Jung's speculations on introversion and extraversion. It is a problem which necessarily poses the question of what is and our relation to what is. Jung's designation of introverted and extraverted types is a product of his peculiar approach to this problem. It is an approach which in turn reveals the influence of his field, psychology, and of the formal intellectual mode of his time. The philosophical question is couched in terms of the role of the subject and object in perception and in terms of a dualistic and predominantly intrapsychic scheme.

The structural model, which is the first of two implicit in Jung's major work on types, largely proceeds by linking introversion with a domain of the psyche. The introverted attitude is a view of objects and situations which results from the interposition of the contents of a particular psychic domain. This conception suggests that the to-be-explained phenomenon called "introversion" is a view of the world which mediates between the occasion of an object or situation and consciousness of it in such a way that there is in some sense less correspondence between these than there is for a second group of people, the *E*s. The view so given or the behavior which may be consequent to it or both are often seen by others as idiosyncratic or whimsical. But in Jung's thinking, the interposed material is itself reflective of a world equally as real, "as much a fact," as is the view and behavior which correspond more to an actual present reality. It is as real, and it is only in appearance idiosyncratic. In fact, by its association with the collective unconscious, the introverted view is said to be expressive of something universal. It is "subjective" in the sense of expressing some more essential aspect of man. With the conceptual linkage given by the structural model, Jung recasts the *I* away from the popular image of him as a withdrawing, somewhat peculiar character. According to this conceptualization, the *I*'s apparently whimsical response is laden with a historical density and a measure of essential truth.

This explication of the structural model will provide guidelines toward the description of introversion in experiential terms. We ask the reader to hold onto the idea of the introverted attitude as a mediated view and to the notion of correspondence, or lack of it as it applies to the perception of an *I*.

It should be clear, however, that while the model or its present explication will provide a set of guidelines, it does not itself directly give us the required experiential terms. We have tried to clarify the difficult notion of the collective unconscious and through it what is meant by the statement that introversion is a "subjective" view. But the clarification leaves the experiential question without resolution. What is the experience of an attitude so given or so determined? What is the introverted experience of the world as a consequence of this particular interposition? We shall demonstrate that these questions remain unanswered even when we turn later from these theoretical models to examine Jung's more "descriptive" writings on introversion. We have guidelines toward the *I*'s world as he experiences it but not yet a description of the thing itself.

Dynamic Model

Explication

One would have hoped that the dynamic model might have completed the picture by characterizing the movement and the laws of movement between the domains and by adding to what is fed into consciousness how it is fed in. This is not quite the case. The structural model even with its own scaffolding leaves questions unanswered: In what way is the subjective view interposed? In what way does the model explain how the two domains are only relatively determinant? Our understanding of the dynamic model is that it puts forth a conceptualization of I/E formally quite distinct from that of the first model. The reason for this will be apparent in the fourth chapter when we employ the explications of the two models as guidelines for the experiential formulation. Let us simply assert for the moment as a point eventually to be demonstrated that this second model, like the first, does point to something in experience. It does represent, although in abstract terms, some essential aspects of the experience of introversion. The primary task here is to explicate the model within this conceptual sphere. Again, the point of departure is the problem of the role of the subject and object in perception.

The dynamic theory, like Freud's, takes energy in a relatively closed system as its model. Jung devotes considerable effort to distinguishing his concept of energy or libido from what he held was Freud's narrower and more specific notion of sexual energy (Jung, 1928). For our purposes, we might note that the similarities are at least as striking as the differences and certainly more easily grasped. In Jung's usage, energy refers to "the intensity of the psychic process. . . . It is a concept denoting intensity or value" (1923, p. 571).

The dynamic or energy model distinguishes introversion and extraversion in terms of the direction of flow of energy between subject and object. Extraversion is defined as a movement of energy from subject to object, while introversion is defined as a movement of energy from object to subject. Direction of flow, for each, is toward the center of "interest" or of "value." The object is of greater value to the E, the subject to the I. It can be readily seen that the second definition of introversion we began with is congruent with this model both in the concept expressed and the language employed. "Libido" is, of course, synonymous for Jung with energy or psychic energy. The definition speaks of movements of energy in two different directions between subject and object.

It is easy to be misled by this definition. That for the I energy moves away from the object does not at all imply lack of interest in the object. Introversion is not the attitude at which a person arrives after he removes energy from the object. The introverted attitude is itself the movement of energy from object to subject. In this, as in the structural model, the object is a central part of the concept of introversion. In the structural model the "contents of the collective unconscious . . . are only released by the operation of the object" (p. 476). The feed-in occurs only on the occasion of attending to an object. Similarly in the present model, the object is essential for the operation of the introverted attitude. It is a movement of energy or value or interest away from the object. The object is a necessary ingredient in any instance of this movement which constitutes in conceptual terms the introverted attitude or view. The term "negative relation to object" in the second definition does not mean that the I fails to relate to objects. It refers to the direction of movement of energy in the model. It is "negative" in the sense of "away from."

The second phrase in the definition, "interest recedes toward the subject," must be understood in a similar fashion. Introversion is not interest in the subject per se or directly or simply. It is a movement of interest toward the subject. Let us take "subject" for the moment to mean "person." Again, this is analogous to the structural model. In that model the *I* does not contemplate directly the collective unconscious in some Buddha-like posture; rather the subjective view occurs as the *I* lives in and relates to objects in the world. In the energy model, similarly, the *I* does not sit encapsulated with his interest focused directly on self. The introverted attitude is an instance of interest moving from moment to moment toward the person, the perceiver.

In addition to the identification of the introverted attitude with the movement of energy in a particular direction, it is also defined within this model in a related way. The introverted attitude is an "abstracting" one. The *I* abstracts or withdraws energy from the object. "The *I*'s attitude to the object is an abstracting one; at bottom he is always facing the problem of how libido can be withdrawn from the object" (p. 412). Again, the object is essential. The energy must be withdrawn from the object. "Interest" is born of or occasioned by the objective situation. Introvertedness again is a process. It is the "abstracting," not the end result of the abstraction that constitutes the introverted attitude in this conceptualization.

Returning for a moment to the example of cold weather: The cold weather is the objective fact which for the *I* is the occasion for energy to flow or to be abstracted from it to the person. There is a movement from the perception or thought of "coldness" to that of "hardening" oneself. And that movement is introversion in this model. For the *E*, interest flows to the objective fact. The idea of wearing a coat is an accommodation to the cold weather.

The model and its application to a differential view of a particular situation is straightforward. This energic concept with its emphasis on the subject and object as two poles or batteries receiving or sending energy in one or the other direction is another guideline toward the description of the experience of introversion. The essential differential aspects of experience referred to by this metaphor, however, remain to be described.

Two points incidental to the main argument may be developed here. The energy model, unlike the structural model, allows Jung to advance the idea of varying degrees of introversion and extraversion from individual to individual. Although energy between subject and object may flow in only one of two directions at a time, the gradient may be variable. Energy flow may vary in "intensity or value" in addition to direction. The degree of intensity or the gradient indicates the "determining power" of the subject or of the object (p. 571). This possibility of variable degrees of an attitude is not extended to include variation within an individual from moment to moment. Jung's concept of neuroticism, which we shall discuss below, does include variation within an individual over greater periods of time as a function of his own development.

The energy model also allows degrees of introvertedness and extravertedness to be thought of as a continuous function; and, at least logically, it allows a point within this continuous function where a person may be equally introverted or extraverted. The gradient may be of any slope. At some point the slope may be zero. In this model the difference between introversion and extraversion is simply a change in the relative "value" of two poles, the subject and the object. There is no discrete and separate domain for each as in the structural model.

Generalizing from these two points, it may be said that the structural model gives the I/E distinction a static and an either/or quality. In contrast, the dynamic model suggests a flexibility both in terms of degree of introvertedness or extravertedness and in terms of a bridge between the two attitudes within an individual setting. The use of energy in a model "allows" such process variables while the use of structure or topography is more amenable to content or thematic variables.

The referent of "subject"

At this point we need to demand of the dynamic model what we demanded of the structural: What is the theoretical referent of "subject" both in the model and in the second definition?

In a context in which he clearly is employing the language of the energy model, Jung states as follows:

In the one case [extraversion] an outward movement of interest toward the object, and in the other [introversion] a movement of interest from the object, toward the subject and his own *psychological processes*. [p. 11, our italics]

Interest moves toward the subject and his own psychological processes. The distinction between object and subject involves, here, at least in part, a distinction between the object itself and the psychological processes occasioned by it. On the occasion of attending to an object, thoughts and feelings appear in consciousness. Interest or value then can move toward the object, or it can move toward the subject's own thoughts and feelings. Jung offers the following statement of this idea:

As a result, the object always possesses for the *I* a lower value; it has secondary importance; occasionally it even represents merely ... the embodiment of an idea in other words, in which however, the idea is the essential factor; or it is the object of a feeling, where, however, the feeling experience is the chief thing, and not the object in its own individuality. [p. 12]

By "psychological process," Jung does not mean by process what would be another possible understanding of the term in this context—the steps by which a person arrives at the thoughts and feelings. He refers rather to the stuff of the process, the thoughts and feelings themselves. To clarify further, he does not refer to the interposing of the subjective view from the collective unconscious. He explicitly states that the *I* is unaware of this "process" (p. 477). As we have suggested earlier, there is little if any articulation between the two models of introversion.

In the energy model *I*s and *E*s do not differ, as they do in the structural model, in that their respective thoughts and feelings arising in consciousness are derived from two different domains. They differ in the direction of movement of energy from subject to object or object to subject, respectively. Added to this is the notion that part of what is meant by "subject" in this model is the thoughts and feelings arising in consciousness on the occasion of the object. "Subject," Jung tells us, refers to both the person and his thoughts and feelings of the moment. In a sense the person and his psychological processes are equated here. This loose equation of "what I am" and "what I am experiencing," although vulnerable to logical analysis, stands up, as we will see later, in an experiential realm of discourse. The suggested equation or linkage is an important one which we shall capitalize on in chapter 4.

Introversion in this model, then, refers to a movement of energy toward what is at the same time self and one's thoughts and feelings of the moment. This movement is focal for the *I*. The *E*, on the other hand, focuses on movement toward the object itself. He is less focused on the thoughts and feelings occasioned by it. This is not to say that he does not have them or that he has less of them in some sense. It is to say that his interest moves from the thoughts and feelings to the object itself.

We have then these additional conceptual guidelines toward the description of introversion in experiential terms. The dynamic model conceives of introversion as a movement of energy (interest or value), and it gives that movement a particular direction. Interest moves toward the subject as person and the subject as that which is being experienced by the person, his thoughts and feelings, on the occasion of a particular objective situation.

The Two Models: Summary

We have explicated the Jungian concept of introversion as it is expressed in these two models. The analysis demonstrates that while both models have the same starting point, the problem of the role of the subject and object in perception, they are more or less independent conceptually. This conclusion does not imply a criticism of Jung's theories. He is not required to have only one model, nor if he proceeds with two models is he obligated to provide articulation between them. In fact it is a major thesis of the present work that Jung invoked two unintegrated models because that which is introverted about an individual is found in two distinct modes of experience. Each model is a depiction of one of the two realms of experience. The peculiarly introverted aspects of each will be described later.

The twoness, in this instance the use of two models, is not a sign of Jung's subservience to the dualistic mode of thought of his day; nor does it bring into question the unity or integrity of the target phenomenon. The formulation of the two models in experiential terms will demonstrate that unity while showing how two distinct models offer here a requisite conceptual maneuverability.

The purpose of the remainder of this chapter is to further clarify the two models by applying them to more of Jung's writings on introversion. Also, we need to establish more explicitly why a formulation in experiential terms remains a residual task despite Jung's opus on I/E. We need to explain how it is that Jung does not leave us with a clear picture of the phenomenon itself (either as it is manifest to others or as it is given in experience). We have from him the conceptual guidelines requisite to locating and grasping the phenomenon directly but we do not have the bridge to the thing itself, the introverted attitude as it appears in experience. These guidelines and the empirical findings of the next chapter, together with an experiential stance to be described, will help effect this merger.

Principle of Opposites

Definition and application

The principle of opposites is basic to Jung's psychology. With it he spells out a dynamic set of relations between the two attitudes as well as between the pairs of psychological functions in his theory of types. Its use is also evident in describing the relationship between archetypal figures in consciousness and in the unconscious. We should now like to examine the principle of opposites as a guideline toward an experiential formulation of introversion.

The principle of opposites states that the two attitudes are polar opposites found in each individual. One pole is located in consciousness, the second in the unconscious. The relation between the two poles, it is postulated, in a function of the degree of "dominance" of the conscious pole. Dominance means a one-sided employment of the conscious attitude, which prevents the expression of the opposite unconscious attitude in consciousness. With minimal dominance, when the unconscious attitude occasionally expresses itself, it does so in a compensatory or complementary way. It adds to or rounds out the conscious attitude in the latter's service. With increasing one-sidedness of the conscious attitude, however, the suppressed unconscious pole has a more opposing or destructive relation to its conscious opposite. It then "irrupts" or intrudes in an "archaic," infantile, and inappropriate manner. This suppression of the other side and its subsequent uncontrollable release is the heart of Jung's conception of neuroticism.

The principle of opposites is then a proposed law which attempts to bring order to our understanding of some of the vicissitudes of consciousness. It posits an unconscious counterpart to whatever attitude or psychological function is dominant, i.e., more generally in consciousness. The counterpart is an attitude or a function which ordinarily does not coexist with its opposite in consciousness. It, however, does "determine" consciousness on occasion by intruding sometimes as a welcome and sometimes as an unwanted guest. The timing frequency, and character of that intrusion is a function of the degree that it is given its due.

The two attitudes I/E are attempts to account for the character of consciousness. The present psychological principle complements them by adding further to the conditions of this accounting. It informs us, for example, that an *I* is not always an *I*. On occasion his attitude may be extraverted, and this extravertedness may have a variable cast. In addition, an *I*'s introvertedness may vary in its one-sidedness, in the pervasiveness of its employment.

These relations between the two attitudes within an individual are not peculiar to the attitudinal distinction of Jung's personality theory. They apply equally to the numerous other aspects of it. The principle of opposites is contributing, for our purposes, less to an understanding of the particularity of introvertedness than to the limits and contingencies of its presence.

The meaning of "opposites": Enantiodromia

The principle of opposites eventually does yield a point which is more relevant to our purposes. Jung borrows a term from an early Greek philosopher, Heraclitus, to express the relationship between two members of any pair of opposites. "Enantiodromia" is translated " 'a running counter to' " (p. 541). This term makes it clear that "opposite" in the principle of opposites is in the sense of opposition. For example, the conscious introverted attitude and the unconscious extraverted attitude in an individual oppose each other. There are different states of tension between them resulting in varying "working" relations from complementarity or servitude to open combat. The members of a given pair of "opposites" then are not necessarily related as opposites in meaning. This suggests that Jung does not consider introversion and extraversion opposites in the sense of antonyms. "Opposites" here is in the sense of opposition. Introversion and extraversion run counter to each other. Each has its own independent mode of operation, and the relationship between the two can be variable.

That Jung does not think of the two attitudes as opposites, like off and on or inside and outside, supports a criticism brought earlier in reference to post-Jungian conceptions of I/E. Simplistic dichotomous or polarized variables cannot capture Jung's notion of I/E even in a theoretical realm. I/E are for him "complexes." They are a set of attitudes not related as antonyms but as alternative ways of seeing, having, or approaching the world. As such the relation between them is more complex and more variable than that between inside and outside.

Conclusion

In a way Jung's interest in I/E is replaced by the principle of opposites. In addition to his consuming fascination with exploring the contents of the collective unconscious, he has a related interest in explicating the relationship between the unconscious and consciousness. Introversion in the structural model is one conception of this relationship; the principle of opposites is an alternative conception. Incidentally, the two notions are not particularly compatible. In the structural model, the introverted attitude is the inter-position of a view from the collective unconscious. According to the principle of opposites, however, what is in the unconscious is not the determining input which constitutes the introverted view. What occasionally irrupts or intrudes from the unconscious, in the case of the *I*, is an extraverted attitude. Of course, Jung's notion of the unconscious is broad enough to house both attitudes and, for that matter, to operate under both conceptions of its relation to consciousness. There is, for example, the distinction mentioned briefly in *Psychological Types* between the personal and the collective unconscious (pp. 615–616). But the two notions of the relationship between consciousness and the unconscious, taken together, crowd each other and render each other less powerful for predictive purposes. If more or less everything is in the unconscious, anything can feed in or intrude.

At any rate, after *Psychological Types* the principle of opposites is repeatedly a central theme while introversion receives little attention and little further conceptual clarification. It is true that I/E are occasionally the particular opposites under discussion, but the focal point is the principle of opposites and, particularly, the intrusive vicissitudes of the unconscious in neurotic development. From their rather special position in Jung's thinking, I/E are relegated to back seats along with such other opposites as thinking/feeling, sensation/ intuition, and masculinity/femininity. Clearly Jung's interest shifted from the study of pervasive and enduring individual differences in orientation to the world to the formulation of a lawful set of dynamic relations between consciousness and the unconscious.

The Later Jung on Introversion

There are several summaries of the history of Jung's use of the term introversion up to and including its use in *Psychological Types* (see, for example, Bash, 1955). The evolution of the concept in his thinking, through *Psychological Types,* may be seen as a mirror of his increasing distance from the psychology of Freud. Initially introversion is a turning of the libido from the object to self-yielding fantasy, a kind of narcissistic cathexis of one's own wish-fulfilling instincts. As such, of course, the term denotes a pathological adjustment. Later, still prior to *Psychological Types,* introversion is associated with thinking or the thinking function and, in a disturbed setting, with paranoia; while extraversion is associated with feeling and hysteria.

Following *Psychological Types,* as noted, I/E receive less central consideration in Jung's writings. There is a short section on them in one of two essays printed in a popular edition (1953), a section which Jung added to an earlier edition of the essay after his completion of *Psychological Types.* The treatment of I/E in the added material contradicts what we have gleaned from the earlier major work in several ways. The only point germane here is that subsequent to *Psychological Types* the stress is already on the principle of opposites. In large part, an *I* is described by depicting what his opposite unconscious attitude of extraversion looks like when it irrupts. There is little direct attention given to the question of what introversion is.

In 1935 Jung delivered the Tavistock Lectures (1968) in which he presented a theory of the structure of the mind. His views had changed considerably since 1923. The ideas of the collective unconscious and of the principle of opposites are dominant. Introversion and extraversion are defined in these terms more exclusively than was the case in *Psychological Types.* Actually, "introversion" and "extraversion" as terms have been replaced by two other terms, "endopsyche" and "ectopsyche." There is only one substantive reference to introversion as the "conscious mind (descending) into the deeper layers of the unconscious psyche" (p. 41). This reference does make it clear that endopsyche and introversion are used interchangeably.

In the later theory "ectopsyche" encompasses the relation between the "external facts" and consciousness; while "endopsyche" is a system of relations between consciousness and the unconscious (p. 11). The four functions which in the earlier typology are vehicles for both of the attitudes are here ectopsychic functions only. The endopsychic operates through different functions. Each of these emphasizes that the endopsyche is a direct expression into consciousness of the collective unconscious and that this expression has an "intrusive," "irrupting," "invading," or "possessing" character (pp. 22–24). The endopsyche or the mechanism of introversion is an instance of the inner life taking hold.

The ideas of the energy model emphasizing the flow of energy from object to subject and the difference in interest or value or weighting are nowhere in sight. In fact, the role of the external object in providing the occasion for the influence of the attitude is minimized, whereas the autonomy of the unconscious and the directness of its expression into consciousness are stressed. Introversion seems to involve a direct line to the unconscious to the exclusion of intercourse with the present objective world.

The structural model is retained but modified drastically. The idea of an interposed subjective view, a kind of subtle posture-determining screen over the world occasioned by an object or situation in the world, gives way to the idea of a more or less autonomous "breaking through" of contents from an "inner" world, a world unshackled from the particular present moment. Further, the character of the contents of this domain now emphasize the dark underside of things: "One has any amount of subjective reactions, but it is not quite becoming to admit these things. . . . These things get definitely painful. That is why we dislike entering the shadow world of the ego" (p. 23). What is left of introversion, if anything, is indistinguishable from Jung's notion of neuroticism. Introversion has come full circle with respect to its association with pathology in Jung's thinking.

In the interim between 1923 and 1935, Jung has explored and "peopled" the collective unconscious. Concomitant with this, the earlier notion of I/E in *Psychological Types* has been lost. Introversion and extraversion are no longer particular and distinct orientations toward the world and one's self in it, postures founded in the necessarily dual aspects of consciousness dealing with the role of the subject or perceiver and the object or perceived. They are no longer distinct approaches to and views of the world which are inherently tied to the objective situation, to a real world event which is the occasion of the respective views. Introversion (or endopsyche) now refers directly to the interface between consciousness and the unconscious.

In brief, as a result of his increasing interest in mapping the collective unconscious, Jung has taken introversion and the introvert with it out of the center of his considerations, thus abandoning the context for further description of the *I*'s experience of the world.

Jung's Descriptions of Introversion

Obfuscating factors

When we turn to Jung's descriptive presentation of introversion, which includes both his portrayal of the appearance of the *I* to others and of the experience of the *I*, we find it very difficult to integrate with the theoretical or conceptual. We want to know, but find it difficult to ascertain, what is the experiential referent of "interposed subjective view," of "turning inward of the libido," of the movement of energy from object to subject, and of other concepts. There is a gap between the theoretical and the descriptive, and we cannot bridge it by direct recourse to his writings.

One reason for this difficulty is simply that Jung does not always make explicit the distinction between the theoretical and the descriptive in his writings. For example, the metaphors which serve as his models of introversion are not labelled as such. But other more serious problems block us from the present goal of extracting from Jung what is descriptive of introversion.

Although the central chapter of *Psychological Types* is over a hundred pages in length, there is little description of the introverted attitude operating in an individual in isolation, as it were. Jung states early that grouping people as *I*s and *E*s "permits no more than a rather general discrimination" (p. 13). It is his observation, hardly to be disputed, that there are "great differences between individuals who nonetheless belong to the same group" (p. 13). In his first complete typological theory he holds that the two attitudes I/E are in all cases expressed through one of four psychological functions. His description, then, is not simply of introvertedness but of introversion as it is manifest through a particular function. In addition, both the attitude and the function may be more or less dominant; and the opposite attitude (or function) in the unconscious, accordingly, may have a particular (more or less neurotic or "inferior") character or relation to the conscious attitude (or function). Of course, all of these ramifications beyond the attitude are part of the formal structure of his typological theory. Our point here is only that they obfuscate the steps from his concepts of introversion to his descriptions of introversion.

There is, finally, more. Jung is aware of the problem of the "personality" of a particular culture in interaction with a particular type. He speaks of a culture collectively as introverted or extraverted, and his descriptions of introversion reflect this interaction. Again, we find it difficult to distinguish the description of introvertedness per se, both as it appears and as it is experienced, from the description of a peculiar mix of introversion molded by a given culture. Jung also stresses his view that an I, for example, looks differently to another I than he does to an E. In all this, Jung intuits and wrestles with many problems that presently receive much attention as methodological issues in personality research and more generally in research in the social sciences: the importance of considering a dimension in interaction with other dimensions, the inseparability of the cultural and sociological from the individual in the study of personality, the problem of observer bias.

We, of course, have no argument with the fact that there is much about an individual which distinguishes him from others. It is not our purpose even to argue with the categories and dynamic relations which Jung feels are particularly invaluable in accounting for individual differences and in describing personality in general. Indeed, to the contrary, one reason we are attracted to the study of introversion is that it has a part in this formidable and intricate typology. The main chapter of *Psychological Types* in which Jung presents the "general description of types" is one of the most compelling descriptions of people in the personality literature or any other literature. One wonders why it is not read more. There is page after page of complexly and richly knit portraits which, as they are brought into the reader's view, become recognizable as and make understandable one or another of his friends, intimates, and colleagues. Our argu-

ment is not with the typology itself with its interwoven consideration of psychological functions, degrees of neuroticism, cultural
context, and the like. We simply maintain that it would have been
possible and desirable to focus more directly on and to explicate
more fully the essential or constitutive features of introversion. Even
if it is only for "a rather general discrimination," we must initially
bracket off other features while we describe it. Until this is accomplished interactions with other dimensions and contextual considerations are more likely to dim than to illuminate an understanding of
the focal phenomenon.

The description

Despite the barriers, let us attempt to extract characteristics of
introversion from *Psychological Types.* The exercise will have the
minimal purpose of illustrating the difficulties just indicated. It will
also demonstrate further how the two models of introversion may be
employed to "explain" these descriptive aspects, i.e., how they
indeed comprise what Jung gives us conceptually of I/E.

Jung states that the *I* appears to others as a "taciturn, impenetrable, often shy" person (p. 413). The impenetrability is emphasized
throughout his description of the various types. The *I* is "inaccessi-
ble" or "hard to understand." This impenetrability or opacity is
acceptable in terms of the idea, in the structural model, of the lack
of correspondence between an objective situation and a subsequent
view of it. But already it is not clear whether Jung believed that these
traits are intrinsically introversion or are an appearance given by the
interaction of introvertedness with a particular culture. Jung states at
various points that the culture of which he is an observer has failed
to recognize the "subjective factor." In a culture where this was not
the case, would the *I* appear less impenetrable? Incidentally, Jung
considered this failing of the culture as just that, as an "error" (p.
473).

When speaking of another characteristic that the *I* displays to
others, Jung explicitly states that the trait is a function of the *I* in
interaction with a particular culture. The *I* is seen in the "generally
accepted extraverted view" (p. 474) as "egotistical" and "egocen-
tric." That the culture has an extraverted point of view does not
mean that only *E*s have this impression of *I*s. The influence of the
particular cultural view is equally "accepted" by *I*s. The implication

is that in a culture with an introverted bent to its view, the *I* would not appear as an egotist.

When we turn to the *I*'s experience as distinguished from his appearance to others the same difficulty arises. There is an ambiguity as to the status of this aspect of introversion. Does feeling like an egotist constitute introvertedness? Jung states, "It is a characteristic peculiarity of the *I* . . . that he tends to *confuse* his ego with his Self, and to exalt his ego. . ." (1923, p. 475, emphasis added). "Self" refers to "the totality of the psyche," the greater part of which is the collective unconscious (p. 540). What is meant here is clear from the structural model. The *I* mistakenly credits to himself that which originates in the collective unconscious. The resultant exalting of his ego is reflected in an enhanced sense of self-importance. But, again, is this tendency to confuse ego with the interposed subjective view a function of introvertedness per se or of the *I*'s embeddedness in a culture which has failed to recognize this view as collective and universal? In sum, we do not know from Jung's writings if a high sense of self-importance is part of the experience of the *I*, and, if it is, whether it is attributable to introvertedness itself, to the influence of the particular extraverted setting, or to their interaction.

This ambiguity is elsewhere bothersome. We mentioned earlier that the *I* is unaware of the origin of his view of things in the collective unconscious. Jung states, "He is just as unaware of the unconscious though thoroughly sound presuppositions of his subjective judgment, as he is of his subjective perceptions" (p. 477). Jung goes on, "In harmony with the style of the times, [the *I*] looks without instead of behind his own consciousness for the answer" (p. 477). He tends to look to the objective world as the origin of his "subjective perceptions." Is that he does so a function of his introvertedness, or is it another confusion or error attributable to the influence of the particular culture in which he finds himself?

Despite these ambiguities in the explication, there are several points that at a later juncture we shall have to try to put together: the issue of the *I*'s awareness of his "subjective perceptions"; the idea that the *I*, perhaps in general, tends to confuse his ego with his Self; and the idea from the energy model that the thought or feeling itself is, to the *I*, of primary importance, while the objective situation occasioning the idea is of secondary value. Of what is the *I* aware; what is the precise focus of his awareness as distinct from that of an *E*; and, more generally, the question we formulated at the outset, what is the experience of "subjective perceptions?" We return to these issues in the fourth chapter.

One other general descriptive point that Jung makes about the *I* has to do with what he terms the "relation of adaptation" (p. 414). This is the difference between introversion and extraversion, "considered biologically." The *I* adapts by concentrating on securing "self-protection," whereas the *E* adapts by "increased fertility." To evidence this biologically based contrast, Jung gives the following descriptions of the *I*: "[The] tendency of the *I* [is] to defend himself from any expenditure of energy directly related to the object, thus consolidating for himself the most secure and impregnable position" (p. 414). Part of the description seems to follow from and clarify the meaning of introversion in the energy model. The *I* does not directly invest his energy in the object. Energy flows from the object to the subject. But there is an additional idea here which we have not encountered before and which suggests something, despite the biological context, about the *I*'s experience of the world and himself in it. Investment in an object is associated by the *I* with a concern with a threat to his security; the *I* is concerned with being in a vulnerable position. Perhaps the example of an I/E difference with which we began has more significance than what we have noted to this point. The *I*'s desire to "harden himself" by not wearing a coat is related to a concern with self-protection. In some way, focusing interest on the subject involves a defensive function. But, once again, it is unclear to what extent this defensive posture is reactive to a particular cultural context—". . . the style of the epoch in which he [the *I*] participates is *against* him. . . . He finds himself in the minority not of course numerically, but from the evidence of his own feeling" (p. 497, our emphasis).

We shall end this section with consideration of Jung's description of the *I*'s relation to the object. Here, again, while Jung's description is variegated and complex, much of it refers to the appearance of the *I* to a particular other in a particular culture (an *E* in an extraverted culture) and to his appearance and experience with increasing one-sidedness of the attitude.

In the second definition of introversion with which we started there is the phrase, "negative relation of subject to object." As we have argued, this refers directly to the energy model, and "negative" describes the direction of movement of energy for the *I*. Introversion is a kind of subtracting of energy from the object. The phrase "negative relation" is not meant to be directly descriptive of the *I* interpersonally. For example, it does not refer to a negativistic or oppositional mode of relating, or to an isolative or disaffiliative mode. The term is part of a metaphor for introversion, energy in a closed system. Once again, the task of locating and describing what this term of the metaphor refers to in the phenomenon of interest is a residual one.

At a point where Jung unambiguously does step clear of the two models, his description of the appearance of the *I* to others varies as a function of the dominance of the introverted attitude. The "milder type" (less dominant conscious attitude) of *I* gives the impression to the other that he, the other, is an object of "indifference" to the *I*. With the "more extreme" type of *I*, the other feels as if he were an object for whom the *I* has some "aversion" (p. 485). In terms of the *I*'s experience of the other, we are told that he "drains" and "disarms" the object, but that he is unaware of his "depreciation" of the object (p. 501). The *I*, then, does not himself experience an indifference or an aversion to the object.

Elsewhere throughout this main descriptive chapter, Jung employs terms such as "defective relation" and "unrelatedness" to describe an *I*'s relation to an object. Here he seems to go beyond the idea of a negative relation in the sense of value or interest moving away from, being drained from, the object. But again the terms are not directly descriptive of introvertedness. The terms refer this time to the structural model. As we have seen, Jung's belief in the dualistic nature of the psyche underlies the structural model. The *I* is unrelated to the external object because the latter is replaced by the subjective object as an image, thought, or feeling from the collective unconscious. It is to this "reality" that the *I* is related. In this sense, he is unrelated to the reality which is the external object. It is clear that Jung does not intend us to believe that it is within the *I*'s experience that he feels unrelated to the external object. He has told us that the *I* looks "without [in front of] his consciousness"; the collective unconscious origins of his thoughts are not part of his experience. What, then, is the peculiarly introverted experience of the other person? Again, a residual question.

Conclusion and summary

If we keep in mind that some, if not most, of these points are descriptive of the *I* in a particular cultural setting only and that some of them are a function of degree of neuroticism, we may conclude this section with a brief sketch. The *I* appears to others as taciturn, shy, and impenetrable. Interpersonally, he seems egotistical and indifferent to the other person. In his own view, the *I* feels self-important. He does not invest directly in objects and indeed would feel vulnerable in doing so. Beyond this sense of vulnerability, which itself may be a function of an interaction with a particular culture, it is not clear what is the experiential concomitant of this lack of direct investment. We are led by the dynamic model to believe that his primary interest is in his own thoughts and feelings occasioned by the object, and that his primary relationship is with his thoughts and feelings. There is some indication from Jung's statements that the *I* is unaware of this interest, and certainly he is unaware that it differentiates him from another class of people.

We have emphasized that much of Jung's description of that which is peculiarly introverted in the *I* is obfuscated by cultural context, degree of neuroticism, particular functions, among other things. We should reemphasize that much of Jung's description of what it feels like to be an *I* indiscriminately intersperses the theoretical with the descriptive, the hypothesized explanation with the to-be-explained.

When we attempt to locate in his descriptions the experience of introversion as distinct from both the formal conceptual definition and from the appearance of the *I* to others, we find terms primarily related to the structural model, "mythological images," "primal possibilities," "unconscious images," "dispositions of the collective unconscious" and various terms with the adjective "subjective." There is little attempt by Jung to define the world as it looks to an *I* outside the frame of reference of these constructs. The terms of the energy model are somewhat less bothersome in that the experiential referents to "energy," "interest," "value," and the like are more immediately apparent. But, we conclude, for the most part Jung's models are his phenomenology.

We have approached Jung's writings with the goal of extracting a more precise description of the phenomenon of introversion. Our bias in this search was that this be done in experiential terms, that the experience characteristic of the *I* be clarified. Jung does make clear that introversion is defined by a particular "attitude," "view," or overriding quality or qualities of consciousness. We take this to mean that introvertedness is an experience or mode of experiencing.

We would like to know what that experience is and to define it in its own terms.

When we turn to the descriptive material we find that the steps from it to the models or vice versa are not explicit. Further, while there is considerable exposition of the appearance of the *I* to others, we find it impossible to sort out that which is characteristic of introversion from that which is attributable to one of the functions, or to a particular degree of neuroticism, or to a particular cultural context. Finally, with regard to material on the experience of an *I*, we find, in addition to these same problems, that much of what is said does not go beyond the language of one of the models. The metaphor serves as the phenomenon. We are not told much about how the world is seen by a person whose view is given by the collective unconscious or precisely what is peculiar to the conscious experience of a person from whom interest moves from object to subject. In chapter 4 we shall attempt to fill in the experience of the *I* utilizing the two models as guidelines.

We feel that the concept of introversion and the I/E distinction represent a seminal, intuitive insight into personality. As we examine introversion from its Jungian beginning, however, we find that on the one hand it has been given a reductive treatment, reified in two models which themselves offer some conceptual clarity but from which we can only gain guidelines toward an understanding of the phenomenon in experience; and, on the other hand, that it has been inflated, given to us only as a product of interactions with variables of psychological "function," of pathology, of cultural context, and the like before the starting point was clear. It seems no wonder that many have been attracted to the concept and that each has found something different there.

Jung was an original and productive thinker and one of our most sensitive observers of the subtle but pervasive individual differences that constitute human personality. But an approach to his work which fails to recognize the contingent nature of his descriptions, or which fails first to identify and explicate his theoretical constructs and then to separate their language from the purely descriptive in his writings, cannot hope to rediscover his insight.

2. Empirical Referents of Introversion

Introduction

We present here the results of a project whose primary aim is to add empirical guidelines to the theoretical ones already described. In this way we hope to give the experiential formulation of introversion a more solid base. To Jung's clinically derived insights we add findings derived from a more controlled but less natural setting.

The material with which we chose to work are stories elicited by the Thematic Apperception Test (Murray, 1936). The choice of the TAT as an instrument has several advantages for our purposes. From the total set of cards one can select a subset which contains immediately recognizable and familiar objects and settings. Thus, as stimuli, the cards are relatively unthreatening. Yet since the pictures elicit a wide variety of story-lines and outcomes, as stimuli they are sufficiently ambiguous. This gives our target population, *I*s and *E*s, an opportunity to reveal through their stories that which is focal and constitutive of their respective worlds. With the TAT, unlike an instrument of a more objectified and predetermined form such as a forced-choice questionnaire, we are not required to include before the fact whatever range of dimensions we suspect to be salient and discriminating. This is the main advantage of the TAT. For us it offered the possibility of making explicit the intuitive consensus about the concept of introversion which we, in the study group mentioned earlier, had been unable to articulate. By utilizing the judgment of the senior member of this group as the independent criterion, we can identify the kinds of I/E differences which constituted the basis for his intuitive judgments.

Other advantages of the choice of the TAT, and other purposes of the project, may be discussed by comparison with a measure of I/E which we employed up to the time of this work. The instrument is a forced-choice paper and pencil test called the Myers-Briggs Type Indicator (M-B) (Myers, 1962). It requires the subject to select one of two or three items of the type: At parties do you (A) sometimes get bored, (B) always have fun? The M-B as an instrument commends itself for its statistical properties and for its inclusion of the Jungian psychological functions. The purpose of the instrument is to locate people with regard to both attitude and functions, and to relate these to various behaviors, life styles, vocations, and abilities associated with them. (For a discussion of the M-B and empirical work involving it, see Stanfiel, 1964, pp. 106–116.)

One of our difficulties with the instrument was that we had come to question strongly whether the concept of introversion implicit in its items really captures the Jungian notion of introversion. It defines the I/E distinction within the inside/outside conceptual frame described in the introduction to chapter 1. In particular it posits that the *I* is oriented to an "inner" world which consists of concepts and ideas; while the *E* is committed to an "outer" world which is replete with people and things. Additionally, it defines the I/E difference by reference to a preferred mode, which for the *I* is said to be reflection and for the *E*, action.

That these definitions do not capture the Jungian concept of introversion is reinforced by our explication of Jung's writings on this topic. In our estimation the distinction is clearly not made between a world of ideas on the one hand and people and things on the other. The distinction must take as its starting point a differential attitude or posture which is prior to the individual's view of ideas, of people, and of things.

In addition to locating and making explicit a construct of introversion closer to Jung's intent, a second purpose of the present project was to generate and test hypotheses relating to I/E differences in behavior and personality. Here again the TAT can overcome some limitations inherent in an instrument like the M-B. We have learned from our research on the Jungian attitudes (Stanfiel, 1964; Bieler, 1966; Shapiro and Alexander, 1969) that simple generalizations, such as the polarities underlying I/E in the M-B, rarely gain clear empirical support. Dichotomies such as concept/people or people/no people do not separate the *I* from the *E*. We have found that to gain empirical support for hypothesized I/E differences we need to specify situational and moderator variables. We must be able to state in what particular situations or contexts an I/E difference will be revealed. The introduction of variables such as neuroticism, task difficulty, and task relevance often reveal I/E relationships that would otherwise remain obscured.

Not only do we feel that the particular polarities with which the M-B defines I/E diverge from Jungian notions, we find that all simple polarities describing I/E fail to find strong empirical support. A forced-choice instrument of the form of the M-B cannot generate the situational or contingent conditions which yield productive hypotheses. We are thus stymied in building a body of experimentally demonstrated situational relations involving I/E.

While Jung's writings do not negate the possibility that there is some I/E difference or differences in an area subtended by a distinction like people/no people, an adequate conceptualization true to the complexity of Jung's thinking must tell us more about the distinction. An adequate formulation must address the following two questions: What is the *I*'s peculiar view of others or of his relations to others? (the experiential question); and under what conditions will the *I* differentially exercise a no-people preference? (the behavioral question).

We have already indicated how an instrument like the TAT, with its ambiguous stimuli and its broad direction to the subject to construct his own story, elicits material likely to answer questions of the first type. Given the open-ended nature of fantasy material, we are free to explore any aspect of the TAT, such as themes, imagery, content, formal elements of language and of story compositions, intrusions of the subject and the like, in an effort to locate attitudinal or experiential I/E differences. The use of the TAT also allows us to search for answers to the second type of question. Since the subject in his stories necessarily describes a course of events or behaviors embedded in a particular situation, we obtain material which may be analyzed as a set of behaviors, outcomes, or preferences surrounded by the requisite discriminating situational variables. This directly solves the problem of generating hypotheses of I/E differences in behavior and/or in other personality dimensions. We can go beyond the simple or generalized hypotheses, which we have seen to have little power, to hypotheses consisting of I/E differences which interact with a particular discriminating condition.

There are two other problems inherent in the use of forced-choice self-description questionnaires for the study of introversion not shared by fantasy techniques. The instrument requires the assumption that the *I* is both willing and able to select his self-description. Jung's statements on the extraverted nature of most Western cultures and its influences on both *I*s and *E*s suggest that the *I* might not be able to do this. A study by Gorlow et al. (1966) also suggests that the *I*, more so than the *E*, cannot or does not disclose himself in a self-description. Gorlow, employing the *Q* sort technique, located the four types combining extraversion and each of the psychological functions but only one of the four introverted types described by Jung. He offers as one possible explanation that "individuals in their self-reports might be reluctant or unable to identify themselves with the introverted side . . . " (p. 117). The TAT, unlike both the Q sort and the questionnaire, confronts the subject with a task which less overtly calls for a self-description. It is, therefore, reasonable to expect less contamination from such factors as cultural or social desirability and response sets.

A final factor in our choice of the TAT was its broad response patterns which offer the opportunity of examining a variety of important personality dimensions within the framework of our intuitive I/E distinction.

There is a possible point of confusion in what we are saying here with regard to the TAT project and a criticism made of Jung in the previous chapter. In chapter 1 we were critical of Jung's inclusion of moderating and contextual considerations, such as neuroticism, function or mode, and culture, in his descriptions of the *I*. We argued that it is possible and necessary, at least initially, to give a description of the essential features of the *I* by bracketing off such considerations. In the present chapter we are choosing to work with the TAT in part because it provides such moderators and contexts. A working model which we employ in our thinking about introversion will clarify this apparent contradiction.

The model holds that there is a core or superordinate concept which is the *sine qua non* of introversion. This core is definable in experiential terms because introversion, Jung states, is an "attitude," i.e., it is an orientation toward or particular view of the world, of one's self in it, and of one's mental processes. It is a general attitudinal approach to all situations. The aspects of experience constituting this core, which we attempt to describe in chapter 4, have predictable effects in behavior. But since I/E is a distinction in experience, we do not expect there to be a behavior across situations which locates all *I*s. This view of introversion requires, then, a second part for our model. In addition to an experiential core existing across situations, there are subsidiary characteristics associated with introversion. These subsidiary characteristics are manifest only in particular situations and only through other personality dimensions or behaviors or both. For example, according to our model we would not expect *I*s in general to be less concerned with affiliation or to have less affiliative behavior than *E*s. But in a particular situation a difference in affiliative behavior between *I*s and *E*s might be revealed. Again, since introversion is an aspect of experience, there is no simple discriminating behavior or behavioral index which locates all *I*s.

With the TAT, then, our primary purpose is to obtain data towards a description of the core of the introverted attitude. We seek features in the stories from which we can infer I/E differences in significant aspects of experience, such as view of and approach to world, self, and own experience. In this regard the TAT offers us fantasy material, the world of an individual projected onto a relatively ambiguous stimulus. Second, with the TAT we hope to locate subsidiary introverted characteristics which can then be experimentally validated by identifying requisite situations in which a behavioral difference or a difference in a second personality dimension or both can be predicted. For this, the TAT is valuable because it provides such moderators and contexts.

Procedure

Ten cards of the Thematic Apperception Test were administered in a group setting. The cards were selected to insure a distribution of the number of stimulus figures in each since relationship to people has traditionally been a central feature of I/E distinctions. Table 1 (p. 56) gives the card numbers, Murray's original descriptions, and the number of stimulus figures in each. Instructions and procedures are taken from McClelland (1962). The cards were individually projected on a screen for 20 seconds. After viewing each card subjects were given five minutes to write a story emphasizing four elements: what led up to the scene, what is happening, the thoughts and feelings of the characters, and the outcome. The subjects were undergraduate students enrolled in an introductory psychology course.

One of us (IEA) experienced in the use of the Jungian typology read each subject's record and eventually labelled it "E," "I," or "uncertain." Those labelled "E" and "I" subsequently served as our independent criterion sort. In reaching a final judgment regarding categorization the record of each subject was reviewed for the number of "E," "I," or "uncertain" stories it contained. On the basis

Table 1. Ten TAT cards employed, with card number, number of stimulus figures and Murray's description.

Card number	Number of figures	Murray's description
1	1	A young boy is contemplating a violin which rests on a table in front of him.
2	many	Country scene: in the foreground is a young woman with books in her hand; in the background a man is working in the fields and an older woman is looking on.
3 BM	1	On the floor against a couch is the huddled form of a boy with his head bowed on his right arm. Beside him on the floor is a revolver.
4	2	A woman is clutching the shoulders of a man whose face and body are averted as if he were trying to pull away from her.
6 BM	2	A short elderly woman stands with her back turned to a tall man. The latter is looking downward with a perplexed expression.
8 BM	many	An adolescent boy looks straight out of the picture. The barrel of a rifle is visible at one side, and in the background is the dim scene of a surgical operation, like a reverie-image.
9 BM	many	Four men in overalls are lying on the grass taking it easy.
10	2	A young woman's head against a man's shoulder.
14	1	The silhouette of a man (or woman) against a bright window. The rest of the picture is totally black.
16	0	Blank card.

of this review, the entire record was then categorized. Typically a record called "I," for example, is either "a clear I throughout" or is basically "I" although two or three stories are "E" or have elements of "E." A record called uncertain has "some E elements and some I elements" or has "I stories with E endings" or the like.

With these records so labelled, we then formed two subject pools.

In the first we required a record categorized as "I" or "E" to be in agreement with an independent assessment gathered from the M-B score for that individual. The first pool, then, consists of the stories of 15 subjects whose total records were judged "I" *and* whose M-B scored "I" points greater than "E" points; and, similarly for the stories of 15 subjects labelled "E." Table 2 (Appendix C) presents a breakdown of this first pool by sex and I/E designation. As can be seen, the sample was somewhat biased in number of males to females, although equally so within "I" and "E" groups. We also obtained, for this pool only, the "function" of each subject as scored by the M-B. Examinations of the functions in combination with I/E on initial I/E operations led us to abandon this further breakdown, since it provided no new information.

The second pool consists of 60 records categorized as "I" or "E" in the manner described previously. Agreement with the M-B, however, is not a condition for inclusion. From the stories of 84 subjects, 30 were judged "E," 44 "I," and 10 "uncertain." The 30 "E" records were combined with a random selection of 30 from the 44 "I" records to make a total sample of 60. Table 2 (Appendix C) presents a breakdown of this second pool by sex and I/E. Again, there are somewhat more males than females. Although agreement with the M-B was not a precondition in determining this second pool, agreement between the judged ratings and the M-B scores is significantly different from chance ($\chi^2 = 15.1, N = 60, p < .01, df = 1$).

This second pool provides the needed sample for cross-validating discriminators emerging from examination of the data from the first sample. It also affords the additional advantage of allowing some estimate of the ways in which the findings are related to the intuitive judgments as distinct from those of the M-B. This may help clarify if and in what ways the evolving notion of introversion is indistinguishable from that which underlies the M-B.

Working with these labelled pools, one of us (KJS) undertook the task of making explicit the bases of the intuitive sort by extracting the I/E differences in the sample. The general procedure followed was to read a number of stories of TATs labelled "I" and "E," identify a difference between them, and frame it in the form of an operation or rule. After obtaining a set of such rules they were applied for purposes of validation to the stories gathered from the subjects in the second pool. This was done blind with regard to criterion label.

Two kinds of operations were formulated. The first, which we will call a "dimension," consists of a statement defined identically across all ten cards. The second type of operation, a "rule," is a statement defined such that it is specific to a particular card. One purpose for framing dimensions as distinct from rules was to test the relationship of theoretically relevant constructs from the personality literature to our criterion I/E sort. Our expectations from this across-card approach were not overly optimistic. As indicated in the introduction, we expected that to discriminate I/E differences with any power we would need to frame an attribute within the situational context offered by a specific stimulus card. A second purpose of this across-card approach, at least in retrospect, was an exploratory one. Occasionally the analysis of a dimension across cards would yield a more powerful split within a particular card. This would then provide a lead for the framing of a rule for that card. Because of this progression, dimensions and rules are in some instances conceptually or thematically related.

Rules are generally in the form: If A and X, score "I," if A and Y, score "E"; if not A, do not score. "A" is a situational variable peculiar to a card. The approach in arriving at rules of this form can be described briefly in two steps.

First, stories told to a single card are read in order to locate all commonalities, either thematic or formal. Once a commonality is found in a sizeable proportion of the stories, variations are sought within the isolated common element. For example, on card 2, a "country scene," a theme common to many stories is that the foreground figure is said to be leaving the background figures. Given this theme, a search is made for variations in the expressed reason for her leaving, in the duration of the separation, or in the presence or absence of feelings expressed by the figure leaving. These variations are checked to determine whether they discriminate between the stories of _I_s and _E_s.

With some exceptions to be noted, the first pool was employed to frame and to provide an initial test of a rule or dimension. As a rough rule of thumb, if the dimension split this pool at a ratio of 2/1 or greater agreements to disagreements with the criterion sort, we proceeded further to validation with the second pool. A more stringent cutoff point was invoked in accepting a rule in the validating stage. A rule had to agree with the criterion at a 3/1 or greater ratio in the predicted direction. It should be clear that a given dimension or rule might attain statistical significance without reaching either of these levels of stringency. These specified rules of thumb are only informal decision strategies.

In the presentation of findings, results are grouped in related clusters. Dimensions and rules conceptually related are presented together and are in turn grouped within topics (see Appendix C, Table 3). Significance levels are given in the text.

Before turning to the presentation of findings, we will describe the actual order in which the work was done. This will give an overview of the methodology and it will also indicate, by outlining results at different points along the way, the basis and direction of certain changes in the procedure and goals of the project.

Much of the work of this project was done over the period of two consecutive summers. In the first summer a number of theoretically relevant variables were tested across cards as were a number of other dimensions generated by a reading of the stories. These were initially formulated and scored with the first pool. Later in the year a cross-validation was attempted by scoring 40 of the 60 records from the second pool. The remaining 20 TATs were left unread. The 40 were obtained by random selection of 20 "I"'s and 20 "E"'s. In this way a batch was left "fresh" for a second round of generating operations which subsequently proved necessary.

Of the 11 dimensions which were formulated and for which validation was sought, 10 of the 11 sorted in the predicted direction and 4 of the 11 retained a 2/1 ratio of agreements to disagreements with the criterion sort. None of them reached the desired 3/1 ratio. All of these dimensions, however, with one exception were scored with a low frequency. Generally, somewhat less than one of ten stories yield scorable instances of a given dimension. Further, internal analysis of the dimensions often demonstrated that one or two of the ten cards elicited the bulk of the scorable instances. In such instances an attempt was made to utilize this information in framing rules to those particular cards.

Also in the first summer we framed 13 rules by card. The results of their validation with the 40 TATs were poor for the "E" part of the rules. For several of the "E" rules or "E" parts of rules, the split was not even in the predicted direction. Results with the "I" part of rules were more encouraging. Of the 11 rules in which a score of "I" was involved, scoring for "I" yielded all but one rule in the predicted direction. Further, four of the 11 reached an approximate 3/1 ratio of agreements to disagreements with the criterion.

An examination of those stories in which intuitive clinical judgment and M-B scores are in disagreement gave additional encouragement with respect to "I" rules. Results are in the predicted direction using clinical judgment rather than the M-B as a criterion when the two are at variance.

Since the nature of introversion was the major point of interest it was decided to concentrate further efforts on generating more rules which would pick out *I*s only. In light of our agreement with Jung that I/E cannot be thought of as antonyms, the constraint that the obverse of an *I* rule must pick out *E*s is unnecessary and unjustified. The second summer was consequently spent in attempting to locate "I" rules to add to the four that had survived the first round. Three such rules were formulated working from that part of the second pool (*N* = 20) not used in earlier validation.

Eventually seven rules were derived which selected *I*s with a 3/1 ratio of agreements to disagreements for both pools combined (*N* = 90). Complete definitions and illustrations of their application are given in Appendix A (pp. 162–165). Brief definitions of each are as follows:

1. Score "I" on card 1 when the object pictured ("violin") is itself seen as interesting or stimulating.
2. Score "I" on card 1 when there is mention of only the figure pictured—no "other" person is brought into the story.
3. Score "I" on card 3 BM when negative affect is associated with the figure and the figure reacts in a self-reliant way.
4. Score "I" on card 3 BM when there is mention of only the figure pictured.
5. Score "I" on card 9 BM when a negative view of the figures or their way of life is expressed; or there is an emphasis on the unpleasantness of the context.
6. Score "I" on card 9 BM when a significant distinction is made between any one or more of the figures.
7. Score "I" on card 14 when the figure is described without allusion to specific others and either there is an indication that the figure has a habit of or comfort in solitude or that the figure is an introspective or "thinking" person.

What does an analysis of these seven rules tell us about the *I*? We have organized the discussion of the concept of introversion emerging from an analysis of these seven rules into two general themes: distance and self.

The Referents

Distance: Rules 2, 4, and 6

At the outset of our work with the stories of *I*s and *E*s it was obvious, even from a casual reading, that there was a striking difference between them in the quality of interpersonal relationships described. A major assertion stemming from this work is that the concept "psychological distance" captures this difference and may be central to all considerations about introversion and extraversion. The *I* consistently demonstrates in his stories a greater sense of distance than does the *E*. We will begin with an elaboration of this sense of distance and present the empirical results relevant to it. We shall leave the path by which we arrived at the concept for subsequent sections.

The present concept of psychological distance is at base a sense of distance between people. It is a quality that an individual feels exists between people, and most poignantly between himself and another person. From this core definition we might expect the *I*'s sense of distance to be manifest in attempts at gaining distance. Thus we might have expected him to include in his stories more instances of the individual leaving another or pushing another away. As we will see, although there are some trends in these directions, the sense of distance is not expressed in this way. That it is not is crucial to an understanding of the concept. We are not dealing with a differentiating aspect of I/E that is motivational or dynamic in character. The *I* is not motivated to gain distance. The sense of distance is inherent in and is a necessary concomitant of some core aspects of the *I*'s experience. This matter will be dealt with at some length in chapter 4. For now, "distance" shall mean that the *I* assumes that there is a greater psychological remove between people than does the *E*. The *I* places individuals at a greater distance from each other than does the *E*.

How is this sense of distance expressed by the *I* in TAT stories? Consistent with our expectation about the ineffectiveness of simple generalized dimensions in discriminating I/E, a single operation of distance defined across cards does not prove to be a powerful sorter. We found, eventually, that the way in which the *I* expressed distance is a function of the number of figures in the stimulus card. When there is only one stimulus figure, the *I* more often than the *E* does not introduce a second person into his story. When there are three or more figures, the *I* more likely emphasizes the differences among the individuals and hence their separateness or apartness. When there are two figures an I/E difference in sense of distance is less apparent. There are some indications that the *I* more often describes a situation where there is no communication between the two individuals. However, this trend, while suggestive, does not attain statistical significance. Having summarized the results with regard to "distance" let us describe more precisely the course of development of this dimension and the rules upon which it is based.

In an initial effort to capture the difference between the two sets of stories, an operation across cards was defined which scored both the theme of psychological distance and a traditional clinical index of distance. Examples of the theme are stories in which the figures are said to live in two different worlds, where there is a "gulf" between them, or where there is an emphasis on the disparity of their points of view. The clinical index of distancing is scored where the subject makes a point of setting his story remotely in time or place or both, i.e., distances himself in relation to the people in the story. Scoring in this manner it was found that the *I* assumes in his fantasy productions a greater psychological distance between people than does the *E* (I = 22, E = 7). Three hundred stories, ten each for thirty subjects, yielded this result. Encouraged by the split, ways were sought to increase the scorable frequency of "distance" indicators.* Two additional scoring criteria were delineated. One included situations in which there is no communication between the figures pictured on the cards. Lack of communication is distinguished from an instance where an attempt at communication fails. The reasoning was that while an assumed apartness or interpersonal distance might be expressed by the absence of communication, abortive attempts at communication suggest that any felt-distance present is not taken for granted but rather is to be changed. Stories were also scored when no mention is made of a second person on a card containing a single figure. Here comfort with aloneness, a sense of the naturalness or completeness of aloneness was thought to be consistent with the notion of an assumed sense of distance from the other.

Results from a new sample with this expanded definition remained encouraging, frequency increased and the *I*s again contrib-

---

*A striking finding which heavily influenced future strategy was that more than two-thirds of the scorable responses occurred on two of the ten cards. This led to the search for card-specific scoring rules.

uted more scorable stories than the Es (I = 59, E =· 32). The frequency of instances increased here to a point where one of every 3.3 "I" stories was scored. When the stories of all three samples (N = 90) were scored with this expanded definition the results remained consistent. The Is provided more than twice as many scorable instances of "distance" than the Es (I = 111, E = 54).

Further work isolated three rules which were card-specific. Two of them were abstracted directly from the operation of distance and a third is related thematically. Two of the rules involve cards with one stimulus figure (cards 1 and 3 BM). For both cards a story is scored "I" when no new figure is introduced beyond the one appearing in the card. Introverted subjects are less likely to create a character than their extraverted counterparts, although both groups are strongly pulled in this direction. On card 1 the split is I = 10, E = 2, p = .03. On card 3 BM the I's stories are scored 17, the E's only 5, p < .01. In his stories to both of these cards the I expresses distance from the other by the omission of any other. There is no indication that the pictured figure is missing someone in the situation. Distance from the other, here aloneness, is simply assumed.

It is important to note that neither of the two cards requires that a second person be introduced in order to create a story. In a sense, the I responds appropriately to the stimulus as presented by not bringing in a second person. For the I, a setting in which an individual is in the exclusive company of himself provides a sufficient setting for a meaningful or complete story. Three other rules dealing with cards with one figure will provide more data on the fantasies of the I given such a stimulus, and hence will allow us to comment further on just what the I experiences in this particular context.

The third of the seven rules is related to the concept of distance although it was not part of the initial operation of distance. The card involved (card 9 BM) is the only one of the three cards with "many" figures which clearly pictures a group scene. This rule scores an emphasis on differences between individuals. The rule scores "I" when "a significant distinction is made between any one or more of the figures" in the group scene of card 9 BM. When applied to the total sample of stories to that card, Is yield 32 scorable instances, Es only 12, p < .01. When given this stimulus of a group scene, the I breaks up the group by making distinctions between individuals. The I less often builds a story in which he takes the group as group. These distinctions place distance between the members. By contrasting them, by emphasizing differences between people, the *I* deemphasizes their commonality and their membership in a coherent entity. Through distinction-making, a clear sense of greater distance between individuals emerges.

The stories scored by this rule may be divided into two subsets. In the first, one figure is described as a nonmember of the group. In the second, one or more significant distinctions are made between a figure or figures within the group. The first kind of story is not as frequent as the second, accounting for only about one-third of the scored instances.

The first kind of story is structured such that one person, presumably the figure with whom the subject identifies, is given some distance from the others. In addition to actual physical distance, he is usually given the psychological distance which is a concomitant of membership in a different social class or stratum. He is most often placed in a higher social stratum than the others. He looks down on the others from a distance. The significant distinction in this first kind of story is primarily a self/others one. These stories much less rarely than those in the second class go on to make further significant distinctions within the "others." It would seem that distance for these *I*s is accompanied by some discomfort with groups.

In the second class of stories however, distance is not a function of nonmembership or of being an outsider. The teller more often assumes the legitimacy of the group but then goes on to make distinctions between its individual members. Distance is assumed within the context of the group. Distinctions are not of a self/others kind, but rather emphasize the difference among all individuals. Here, the bases of the assumed-distance are the distinctions that lie between individuals.

It should be clear that these three rules and the related dimension described earlier are not themselves direct measures of an expressed feeling of interpersonal distance. Rather, the notion of assumed or felt-distance makes sense of what the *I*s do in their stories that distinguish them from stories of the *E*s. The notion of distance is for the moment part of a construct of introversion arising from this project. In chapter 4 this construct and the particular rules upon which it is built will be taken as guidelines for the experiential formulation. At that point felt-distance will be described more fully and precisely and its place shown within that formulation.

Traditional referents

Affiliation or sociability. Before presenting the second part of our construct of introversion, we will present the results of some other comparisons made at the same time. We began by investigating several personality variables which we felt might be relevant to introversion. Among the variables we were particularly interested in was affiliation, since some notion of affiliation, sociability, or sociophilia is the central construct in most measures of I/E. Additionally, in everyday usage I/E is rendered roughly as a liking or not liking of people. Despite the apparent promise, we discovered no I/E difference in affiliative or sociophilic dimensions in these fantasy productions. We will describe the particular operations which we employed.

Shipley and Veroff (1962) score instances of a concern with establishing, maintaining, or restoring a positive affective relationship as an expression of affiliation motivation. Using this definition, instances of affiliative imagery are not significantly different in the stories of Es than in those of Is, although there is a trend for Es to give more scorable responses (E = 31, I = 20, p = .14). When a refinement of this measure of affiliation introduced by Atkinson et al. (1954) is applied, namely a distinction between approach and deprivation affiliation, it fails to increase the I/E difference. The former is defined roughly as an approach to people that is motivated by warmth of feeling with people; the latter is defined roughly as an approach to people motivated by an attempt to avoid noxious states such as loneliness. Although internal analysis of affiliative imagery by card reveals that one or two cards elicit a disproportionate number of instances of scorable imagery, we were unable to frame a satisfactory rule for either card.

We also studied affiliation by framing an operation of disaffiliation, i.e., instances where the subject goes out of his way to disclaim affiliative interests or motives. We defined as "no relation" an instance where a subject denied a close relation by describing two or more people as meeting only accidentally, incidentally, casually, or professionally, like employer/employee or messenger/message receiver. This operation also fails to discriminate between I and E stories.

These results taken together indicate that fantasy concerning affiliation is not a powerful discriminator of introversion and extraversion for our criterion sort. Data from the two TAT measures of affiliation and from our operation of disaffiliation suggest that the affiliative or sociophilic dimension is not central to our implicit construct of introversion.

Now let us report briefly the investigation of two other personality dimensions which factor analytic studies suggest are relevant to I/E. The first, need for achievement, described by Atkinson (1958), failed to differentiate stories of *I*s and *E*s in our first pool of subjects. We had reasoned that since introversion was shown to be related to a concern with agency (effectiveness, instrumentality), with enhancement of self, or with both, this might result in more achievement imagery.

Similarly, a measure of power motivation developed by Veroff (1957) had little success in separating our sample. Our speculation about power, again suggested by factor analytic studies, had been that *I*s might show a greater tendency to describe relationships between people in terms of dominance and manipulation and that this might be reflected in more imagery involved with power and relative stature. We found no evidence to substantiate this conjecture.

Personal interaction variables. Investigating the affiliative dimension we had asked an essentially quantitative question involving the number of interpersonal relationships and the degree of focus on them. At that point, before we were yet on to a notion of distance we asked one further question of kind or mode of relation or interaction. Given that a story involves a relation between two or more people, in what ways do *I*s and *E*s consistently differ in the kind of interaction portrayed? The analysis of personal interaction variables may be seen also, in retrospect, as an attempt to clarify I/E differences in the description of dyads, since the cards with two stimulus figures, as previously mentioned, yield no rule for a sense of distance.

The findings with these variables are surprisingly unproductive. We can locate no clear difference, in the stories of *I*s and *E*s, in the kind of interaction described. The pushes and pulls of personal interactions and the ways in which they are expressed do not reveal a characteristically introverted mode of interaction. Detailed results are presented in Appendix B. Here we will review our approach to the question of mode of interaction.

Karen Horney's descriptions of neurotic styles provide a framework of three basic modes of relation to others, moving toward, moving away, and moving against (1937). We constructed several measures to get at possible I/E differences in the kinds of interactions which may be organized within these categories. Most of the findings yield no more than trends, and many of these no longer remain after attempts to cross-validate them. It is clear that we cannot describe the *I* reliably in terms of the personal interactions which we investigated. There are, however, suggestive indications in the results that a particular flavor distinguishes the interactions described by *I*s from those of *E*s. It is a distinction consistent with the trend we found in measures of affiliation. Along with the tendency for *I*s to include less affiliative or sociable material in their fantasies, we can add the finding that interactions described by *I*s have a more antisocial or mildly misanthropic tinge. There are trends for the figures described by the *I* to do more moving against; while the *E*'s figures do more moving toward. An *I* tends to portray a relation as more asymmetrical and exploitative; the *E* as more mutual, cooperative, and empathic. The *I*'s figures more often blame the other; the *E*'s more often blame themselves. Again, all of these results constitute only a consistent coloring. Clearly I/E differences in dyadic situations are more complex, and hence harder to tease out, than are I/E differences in situations where there is either one or many figures.

At this point, given the consistent thematic tinge of these results and yet their equally consistent lack of power as I/E sorters, we were led to make a distinction between mode of interaction and a more static and assumed quality of being with the other which pervades the *I*'s stories. This distinction allowed us to formulate the concept of psychological distance, framed in the various ways we have described.

Affect: Rule 5. One other approach which we took in our effort to isolate I/E differences in the area of interpersonal relations was an investigation of expression of affect. We were led to this by suggestions in the literature that negative affect, particularly depression, is a likely concomitant of the introverted attitude.

We noted the number of affect words used by *I*s and *E*s in their stories and scored each either as an expression of positive or negative affect. "Happy," "enjoy," "feeling good," and the like we counted as positive, and "sad," "distressed," "lonely," and the like as negative affect words. "Anger" and related affect words were excluded as we had examined them earlier under the personal interaction variable "moving against," without success.

The data were analyzed by examining I/E differences in the use of positive and negative affect words for groups of cards containing the same number of stimulus figures. Cards 1, 3 BM, and 14 formed a group with one figure, cards 6 BM and 10 a unit with two figures, and cards 2 and 9 BM one with many figures. Results are presented in Table 4 (Appendix C, pp. 169–70). When all cards are combined, there is a trend for Is to use more negative to positive affect words than do Es ($p = .12$ for 210 stories). For particular groups, Es project more positive to negative affect than do Is on the group of cards with two figures ($p = .03$ for 60 stories) and a similar trend in the same direction exists in the group of cards with many figures ($p = .14$ for 60 stories). There is also a trend for Is to project more positive than negative affect relative to Es on a group with one figure ($p = .23$ for 90 stories). While only one of these results is statistically significant, they at least suggest that Es relative to Is may have more positive associations to or are more comfortable with a situation in which there is more than one person and Is may be more comfortable in a situation in which they are alone. This last is consistent with the highly significant finding that Is less often than Es introduce a second person into stories told to cards with one figure. Such a situation is complete in itself for the I.

One of our seven rules is a refinement of this work with affect words. We score a story "I," told to card 9 BM, in which a negative view of the figures or of their way of life is expressed or a story in which there is an emphasis on the unpleasantness of the context (Rule 5–I = 30, E = 9, $p < .01$). We earlier described a rule to this same card from which we inferred that the I emphasizes the differences between individuals in their perception of a group. Here we can add that to the extent that the I perceives a group as a group he tends to associate it with a negative way of life or an unpleasant context.

Self: Rules 1, 3, 7

Three of the seven rules constitute the second part of the construct of introversion which emerges from this project. Each of them identifies some peculiarly introverted view of self, self-concern, or the like. Several findings discussed earlier led us to look for I/E differences related to aspects of self. The two rules about groups both suggest a difficulty for the I in accepting group identification and a focus on individual identity. Rules 2 and 4 also point to a comfort with and completeness of the individual when alone and perhaps accompany a peculiar view of self as isolatable in fantasy. In addition, of course, Jung's definitions of introversion point in this direction: the *I* is oriented to the subjective. What does this mean for the *I*'s view of himself and of his position in the world which might surface in his TAT stories?

Finding aspects of these stories from which we could infer something about self is not an easy task. Actual self-reference, direct allusion by the storyteller to himself, is rare. Aspects of stories from which potential measures of relevant dimensions like degree of self-awareness could be constructed are even more difficult to locate.

Using a more thematic approach, we were able to formulate a dimension across cards that was eventually somewhat fruitful. Stories about going off to make one's fortune, or about career choice and ambitions, are fairly common. These kinds of themes, broadly about "bettering oneself," led us to a definition of self-development as a more visible aspect of concern with self. However, it became clear immediately that a broad and general definition of concern with self-development gave no I/E split. An analysis of stories told to the two cards which elicit this theme most strongly (cards 2 and 8 BM) demonstrated that several subthemes needed to be sorted out before an I/E difference could emerge.

We then framed and tested an operation of concern with self which excluded the contaminating subthemes. We scored self-concern when it is judged to be an end in itself. This theme is inferred from stories in which a character inspects the self through consideration of changes in self, of growth of self, and of the question of the fittedness of self. By this last is meant a concern with the question: What are my interests, preferences, strengths, idiosyncracies? What is this peculiar self fitted to be?

We distinguish this theme of self-concern from the following three subthemes: (1) achievement where it, at base, reflects a concern with helping others, or with status, or with impact on others, or with emulation; (2) autonomy where the concern with autonomy does not also address the problem of what possible direction the self once freed prefers to go and is fitted to go; (3) self-development where it is not an end in itself but rather is in the service of a focal concern with helping, being close to, or having impact on others. Again, the theme of self-concern which we scored has a more introspective quality and is more an end in itself. There is a distinct sense of a searching and inspecting of the self.

The results of scoring this operation in the two samples across cards indicate that it approaches an index of self-concern which is more often found in an *I*'s story (I = 20, E = 5, $p < .01$; I = 13, E = 7, $p = .25$). With this moderately successful dimension, we turned to rules by card to find more powerful and more reliable I/E sorters.

The first of the three rules which we fit under the heading of "self" is a rule to card 1 (Rule 1—I = 15, E = 3, $p < .01$). This card presents the subject with a picture of a boy and a violin. The rule scores a story "I" in which the "object pictured (the violin) is itself seen as interesting or stimulating." In general, stories told to this card typically emphasize the theme of achievement, the conflict between work and play, or the working out of a relation to a significant other, particularly over the issue of authority. The story of an *I* less often deals with these themes. The *I*'s story focuses more directly and more exclusively on the value one object has for engaging the self.

We have seen from Rule 2 that *I*s less often introduce a second person in their stories to this card. The present rule tells us more about what occurs in this unpeopled situation. There is comfort for the *I* in having the figure simply concentrate on the object. The unpeopled situation which appears to be incomplete for the *E* is filled for the *I* by this absorption in the object.

The direct confrontation between boy and violin as a focus of the *I*'s story reinforces a point which earlier findings implied. The *I* is not withdrawn either from the world of persons or of things. The striking sense of distance which he feels does not occur in the context of an individual who is "removed," or fanciful or, in even its broadest sense, autistic. We infer this from the fact that the focus of the *I*'s story is about a direct meeting of a person with something else in the world. We infer it also from the fact that the *I*, in describing this meeting, is focusing on what is the immediate task-demand of the stimulus, a boy facing a violin. The *I*'s story is a product of a direct and appropriate "meeting" of a stimulus situation. Hence the *I* does confront the world directly.

What does this rule tell us about the introverted self? The meeting of the boy and the violin is the occasion of the boy's thoughts and feelings. The object stimulates these thoughts and feelings. The tone of this moment of stimulation is given in the *I*'s stories by the figure's fascination with the object. He approaches it and wonders at it. It is an aesthetically beautiful object, a complex piece of machinery, or a mysterious producer of beautiful music. The moment of stimulation is an absorbing and enrichening moment for the *I*. What is being enriched are the boy's own thoughts and feelings. It is an instance of stimulation of the self or of growth of self. The meeting with the object is an occasion of self-growth as an end in itself.

We have condensed much information about the *I* derived from this rule. In the final chapter we shall connect these points with the theoretical guidelines provided in chapter 1 and with the development of the experiential formulation of introversion. Two questions in particular will need to be clarified at that time: What is the relationship between this absorbing and stimulating confrontation of objects and the sense of distance; and is a person as distinct from a thing sometimes the object of stimulation in this same way for the *I*?

The second rule under the heading "self" is an operation applied to card 14 (Rule 7—I = 18, E = 6, $p < .01$). Stories to this card by all subjects mention only one person considerably more often than not. This omission of mention of a second person does not discriminate *I*s from *E*s. One feature of this card which distinguishes it from the two cards for which this "no mention" rule did discriminate is that there is no obvious additional object or thing in this card. There is only the one figure. But for whatever reason, this card, a "silhouette of a man against a bright window," makes a strong demand for a story of a person in solitude.

Only when we require, in addition to no mention of a second person, a story in which there is "an indication of a habit of or a comfort with or a pleasure in solitude; or indication that the figure is an introspective or 'thinking' person" does the operation pick out the stories of *I*s. Given a stimulus card without a second person and without an object in which to become engaged, the *I* makes one of these related attributions to the figure (see examples, Appendix A, Rule 7). The *I*'s response does not include excuses for solitude. The person is less likely forced to put in an "all-nighter" to catch up on his studies or disturbed by a late party next door. The stories of *I*s reveal a comfort with the exclusive company of oneself or one's thoughts and feelings. Being alone is something the *I* does comfortably from time to time given an appropriate situation. The attributions to the solitary figure reveal a sense of comfort with the exclusive company of oneself. In some situations an *I* is more comfortable than an *E* with what Singer terms an "internal focus" (1966).

The third rule concerning "self" involves card 3 BM (Rule 3—I = 24, E = 9, $p < .01$). A large majority of stories to this card begin with a description of the huddled figure in a stressful or negative situation. This is in accord with Henry's description of the manifest stimulus demand of the card, "the figure is in a situation of a negative character calling for some explanation" (p. 243, 1956). We found no discernible I/E differences in whether the stories described a "tough spot" or in its particulars; nor did we find I/E differences in the events leading up to the negative situation. *Is* do differ from others, however, in the modes by which their characters seek to resolve the problem. The rule states that a story is scored "I" if the figure is in a negative situation and is "self-reliant" in his or her mode of attempted resolution of the difficulty.

In using the term "self-reliant" we are emphasizing only the objects upon which one may rely, the self or the other. Despite the usual connotation, we do not mean to imply by self-reliance a greater effectiveness in resolving a problem. Obviously, a person can rely on self and be relatively incompetent; and, conversely, a person can be skillfully discriminating in his reliance only on highly competent others. On the other hand, self-reliance is not simply a turning away from others. It is a turning toward the self in a positive or active way and as such is not escapist. A story in which the figure "stays in his room" or escapes into daydreaming is not an "I" story. For *Is*, turning toward the self is the preferred means of actually attempting to resolve the problem.

One final qualification, self-reliance does not necessarily imply a difference in the felt locus of responsibility. If the figure in the tough situation calls in another person, he may feel, nonetheless, that he himself is responsible for the resolution of the problem by taking this initiative. While the "self-reliant" person presumably feels self-responsible, "other-reliance" may also be accompanied by a feeling of the self as the locus of responsibility. Again, self-reliance here refers only to the particular object upon whom one relies in seeking a resolution to the "tough spot."

The demands of a stressful situation are a requisite condition for this preferential difference in mode of resolution-seeking. Given stress, the *I*, turns more to self than does the *E*. This finding that the *I*, responding to the stimulus of a person alone in a stressful situation, portrays that person turning toward the self to seek resolution has at least two important implications. First, we take the turning toward the self to imply that the *I*, given a stressful situation, is more inclined than an *E* to have recourse to his own thoughts or feelings or "experience." The *I* prefers to evaluate and to seek solutions for the problem in this way. It is his preferred first step in seeking a resolution.

A second implication of this rule represents an addition to our findings on affiliation. While we have presented results suggesting that affiliation may not be a general I/E discriminator, this rule suggests that stress is a particular situation where *I*s are less affiliative than *E*s. The stressful situation makes a demand on *I*s in response to which a self-reliant preference is manifested. The self-reliant mode of seeking a resolution is one which excludes other people. We have tested this implication in an independent study which we shall briefly review below.

We began this section with an exploratory operation across cards, the theme of which was self-development or self-concern as an end in itself. It received directional support and pointed the way to search for rules by card. We found three such rules which significantly sort the combined criterion pools. From these, we derived several notions about the *I* and self. Given the appropriate setting, *I*s are more likely than *E*s to stimulate their own thoughts and feelings by directly confronting an object in the world. The *I*, in appropriate circumstances, is more comfortable than the *E* with his own exclusive company and his own thoughts and feelings. He does not "excuse" his solitude. Finally, in a stressful situation, the *I*'s preferred mode of seeking resolution is by recourse to himself, to his own "experience."

The Relationship Between I/E, Affiliation, and Anxiety

Let us now turn to a study designed to investigate our hypothesis that the *I*'s resort is to "self" when in a stressful situation (Shapiro and Alexander, 1969). The hypothesis was derived from Rule 3 generated from stories told to card 3 BM, which pictures a single figure usually seen in distress.

The main finding of the study was a predicted interaction between I/E and anxiety on a measure of affiliation. That is, *I*s are less affiliative than *E*s only when in stress. Following Schachter (1959), anxiety was induced by threat of electrical shock and affiliation was measured by the choice to be alone or with others during a waiting period prior to being shocked. We found that anxious *I*s have less desire to affiliate than do either anxious or nonanxious *E*s, while nonanxious *I*s and *E*s do not differ in degree of affiliative desire.

In our examination of measures of affiliation across cards reported earlier, we learned nothing about differences in I/E performance. However, the rule derived from card 3 BM pointed to the fact that stress might be the critical variable in the affiliative choices of *I*s and *E*s. We decided to test this directly. Our rule suggests that an *I*'s reaction to a stressful situation precludes affiliation in that situation. The *I* is more self-reliant in an anxious situation and thus handles the problem alone.

It should be clear that this study does not provide a direct validation of this rule in that we did not employ it or the other rules to select subjects for this study. They were selected by performance on the Myers-Briggs Type Indicator. However, the rule directly and accurately helps us to generate the particular condition within which a predicted I/E relation to affiliation could be expected.

A second result of this study adds evidence to the finding that in fantasy a sense of distance is characteristic of an *I*'s relation to another. Those subjects who made an affiliative choice subsequently spent a few moments together with others. Afterwards they were asked to respond to measures concerned with their perceptions of these others. One of the measures asked the subject to rate his involvement in the group in terms of felt-closeness or -distance from others in the group. In the high anxiety condition, *I*s indicated more felt-distance than did *E*s ($N = 18$, $p < .01$). Thus even when *I*s chose an affiliative response to stress they felt more "distance" from the others than did *E*s.

We should now like to examine the implications of this study for our general conception of introversion.

1. The major finding that a measure of affiliation is related negatively to introversion only in a circumscribed situation supports our position that a conception of introversion which equates it with or even centers it on the sociophilic or affiliative dimension is misleading.

The affiliative dimension is neither focal nor definitive with respect to introversion.

2. The study also supports our point of view that gross generalizations about I/E fail to get at the power of these attributes to predict differences in behavior. To obtain confirmation of predicted

empirical relations between I/E and a second dimension, we need to specify a particular situation within which a difference will be manifest.

3. The study underlines the distinction between the two kinds of I/E differences suggested in our working model at the beginning of this chapter. The first is represented by the interactional finding involving I/E, affiliation, and anxiety. It is an expressed preferential behavioral concomitant of the introverted attitude in interaction with a specific situational variable. Although situationally limited, in that it is reflected in a behavioral choice, it is a difference clearly visible to others. The second kind of I/E difference for which support is gained is represented by the distinction, felt-closeness/felt-distance. This class of difference approximates more closely what is implied by Jung's notion of attitude. While an attitude or orientation or posture may be reflected in behavior, it is at base a distinction in kind of experience or in experience itself. In stating that a person typically feels distant from the other, we are commenting on his attitude to the world, on how he is in the world. He may or may not indicate this aspect of his experience in his behavior to the other. This distinction we hope will clarify further the kind of formulation of introversion to be developed in the fourth chapter.

The Generality of the Seven "I" Rules

To return to the rules derived from fantasy productions, the generality of our findings is subject to the limitations imposed by the criterion sort since it is based on the judgments of one person. These limitations are, we think, offset by his experience with the Jungian typology and the statistically significant agreement of his judgment with at least one other measure of I/E in the literature. However, our choice of procedure was dictated by the wish to make explicit what we felt was valuable on an implicit and intuitive level. We were not concerned with what is consensual about introversion. If we were, we could have used the criterion sorts of Jungian-trained judges, a feasible and acceptable alternative mode of procedure.

A second possible limiting source is related to the problem of drawing inferences about individuals from their fantasy productions, in this instance from stories told to TAT cards. There are discussions in the literature of the assumptions involved in the TAT as well as a large body of relevant empirical knowledge (Murstein, 1965). Prediction of behavior on the basis of various TAT measures is difficult although there have been notable successes and a number of methodological and conceptual advances toward this end. However, this same literature suggests that inferences about attitudes, beliefs, views of self and others, and the like, which are our central concern in this work, are generally less problematic than are behavioral predictions.

In addition to these general considerations the storytelling task with which we worked may present particular difficulties for the study of introversion and extraversion. There is considerable "demand" in the structure of the task and in the stimuli themselves for a subject to focus on relations between people. *I*s and *E*s may differ in their feelings about this demand in ways which would yield I/E differences peculiar only to this set of circumstances. If, for example, the TAT is a task with which *E*s are more comfortable than are *I*s, any differences in the protocols from which rules are subsequently derived may be influenced by the variable, "task-comfort." To the extent that they are, inferences from these rules may be limited in generality.

In this same vein, the setting of the task may also introduce a bias. The stories were obtained in a group administration and the number of people in the test-taking setting may be a situational variable that has relevance for I/E. *I*s, for example, may be more inhibited or more negative than *E*s in this situation. Of course, an individual administration also would introduce a peculiar bias for *E*s and *I*s. Effects of this situational variable could be tested by validating the rules and dimensions derived from the present group administered protocols with another TAT sample administered individually.

In terms of the inferences which we actually drew, the rules and dimensions vary in the degree of confidence they afford us. Of course, the inferences, or at least some of them, are experimentally testable. But, aside from this highly desirable form of confirmation, the inferences about introversion as they stand vary in the degree of certainty with which a discriminating condition is identifiable. For example, what is the requisite discriminating condition necessary to obtain the "negative view" of the group in card 9 BM scored in Rule 5? Is it simply any group scene or must an inference about the *I*'s peculiar affective association to "groups" require that the group be pictured lying prone, as this one is? Unfortunately, the card involving this rule is the only one of the ten that plainly confronts the subject with a group. For this reason we cannot check whether a group in some other setting or posture would produce the same discriminating *I* story.

The discriminating condition in a rule like the "self-reliance" rule (Rule 3) is clearer, since the operation itself includes a commonality within stories which then produces the discriminating variation. Given stress, *I*s differ from *E*s in mode of resolution. A rule like the "no mention" rule (Rules 2 and 4) offers a different kind of check on the discriminating condition. It occurs on two different cards each of which has one stimulus figure and object but does not occur on a card with one stimulus figure and no other object. The discriminating condition is then clear.

The Seven "I" Rules: Some Further Considerations

A major part of this chapter has involved the description of seven rules which discriminate the stories of *I*s. In this section some remarks about their sorting power and distribution and about the fact that these rules locate *I*s only are in order.

Each of the seven rules picks out between one-third and two-thirds of the *I*s in the sample (with the exception that Rule 2 picks out only slightly more than one of five "I" stories). They do so while retaining from a 3/1 to a 5/1 ratio of agreements to disagreements with the criterion sort. There are two exceptions here—Rule 6 and, interestingly, Rule 3, the rule from which we took the hypothesis for the study reviewed above. These two have a slightly greater than 2.5/1 ratio.

A second piece of data involves the fact that three of the ten cards provided stimuli for six of the seven rules. In Table 5 (Appendix C) we present a breakdown of the overlapping and nonoverlapping instances of each of the three pairs of rules drawn from the same card. These data indicate, in each case, that, while there is some overlap, each rule by itself picks out a respectable part of the *I*s in the samples. In addition, in each case, the two members of a pair are more or less conceptually independent of each other in that they point to different aspects of the stories elicited by the common card.

In Table 6 (Appendix C), we have presented breakdowns of each of the seven rules by sex. For each of the seven rules the relative frequency of instances scored is strikingly similar for males and for females, with the exception of Rule 7. Additionally, on Rule 7, females are less clearly sorted in agreement with the criterion. The number of false positives is high. Interestingly, for the males this rule provides the best split. Rules 5 and 6, on the other hand, provide the poorest splits for the males while they are among the best splitting and most frequently scored rules for females. Rules 5 and 6 are both taken from stories told to the "group" card; Rule 7 comes from one of the cards with one stimulus figure.

It is difficult to say what this tells us except that we might better predict introverted behavior when we operate with females in a group situation and males in a solitary situation. Our study on I/E, anxiety and affiliation also suggests or at least leaves open the possibility that we may have a sex difference in the area of introversion on our hands. In that study the predicted I/E difference in affiliation for females did not hold. Although there were clear and demonstrable reasons why the study did not provide a test of this prediction for females,* it may also be true that female introversion at the college age is reflected differently from introversion in their male age mates.

Turning to the fact that these rules measure introversion only, we began this project with the intent of defining operations that would pick out both *I*s and *E*s. We have had considerably more difficulty with the latter; and, as reported, concentrated on the search for introverted operations as these began to emerge. One possible explanation for the one-sidedness of our difficulties may lie in the one-sidedness of the senior author's interest in introversion, an "attitude" which he purports to possess. We add this as another possible limitation or bias of our findings, since Jung's writings would suggest that such a person might be relatively insensitive to the extraverted aspects of the stories and, hence, unable to isolate and define "E" rules.

A second possible explanation follows if we conceive of introversion as a complex characteristic of personality which an individual must realize, perhaps by stages. It may be, then, that it is difficult for people to realize their introvertedness, perhaps particularly difficult

---

*In particular the reasons were related to the power of the manipulation for females and their failure to meet preconditions for the affiliation choice.

in most Western cultures which according to Jung are extraverted, and perhaps particularly difficult for people at the age of those in these samples. It is our impression, for example, that there are several aspects of the experience of introversion which individuals come to tolerate or "allow" only in their young adult or later years. Why this may be the case will, we hope, be clearer in the final chapter.

3. The Problem of Experience: A Phenomenological Description

Introduction

In the following chapters we have the final task of formulating introversion in experiential terms. For this we shall require a set of aspects of the introverted experience which will have some claim to being comprehensive, general, and requisite. They should be features constitutive of introversion. At the same time, they must be embedded in a description which allows, or even compels, the reader to know immediately, unambiguously, and in as full-bodied a way as possible the phenomenon to which they point. The sources of this descriptive formulation are the theoretical notions of Jung presented in chapter 1, the empirical findings reported in chapter 2, and, in addition, our own experience. In this last there is both our "professional" experience, the results of our discussions with each other and with others over a number of years, and our personal experience.

Between these sources and the eventual formulation is the method of moving from one to the other. Before beginning the description of the world of the *I*, we shall indicate this method briefly. We offer this way of proceeding as one generally applicable to problems in personality. It is based on some readings in phenomenology and phenomenological psychology, and draws particularly on the work of Eugene Gendlin. As we stated earlier we are relying heavily on a demonstration of its use to present the method. While discussions of experiential methods and the need for them are numerous, full-scale investigations employing these methods are a relative rarity. Also, that part of the method which may be different than that described in other discussions is readily set forth.

We have noted that our studies of the theoretical writings, the various inventories and measures, and the experimental work on introversion forcibly raised for us the question of how to proceed in personality. We have already discussed critically the problems peculiar to this topic, particularly under the heading, "the problem of introversion." But it is clear from another point of view that much of the problem of introversion is not at all peculiar to this phenomenon or to the history of its investigation, as long and complex as it is. The questions of how to proceed, what is an instance of a problem in personality, and what constitutes saying something about it are general ones which emerge from a critical look at traditional methods.

Roughly speaking, there seem to be three predominant ways of proceeding in psychology: by constructing a model, usually a mechanistic or physical system, which mimics some properties of the phenomenon; by building an empirical network of relationships of the phenomenon under study with other variables; or by delineating the genesis or development of the phenomenon. A difficulty common to all of these approaches is the problem of definition. Each way of proceeding defines the target phenomenon in a different way. Each differs from the others in what it assumes constitutes a definition or conception of the variable of interest. In consequence, different investigators often are studying different phenomena under the same name. This certainly has been the case in the history of work on the Jungian attitudes.

The problem of definition is, however, not only that of finding and maintaining a common starting point. It is also the dangerous hurdle of reduction, of losing the target phenomenon through the way we attempt to fix it. All too often we can research it, work with it, or "define" it in such a way that the phenomenon is left behind, so that we never really contact it, let alone say what it is. One result of this is that there is created through the manner of our approach a discontinuity between research and application, between the mode of scientific inquiry and the life it seeks to know. The dilemma is in how to translate meaningful psychological problems, which involve a certain style of perceiving, of relating to, or acting in the world (Merleau-Ponty, 1962, pp. 153, 183, 209 and elsewhere) into the constraints dictated by our methods and then to retranslate our analogies, measures, operations, developmental sequences back into a practical, felt or embodied understanding of the phenomenon.

It is clear that an analogy to a phenomenon, such as a physical model, is not the thing itself as we meet it in everyday life. Nor is a measure or operation of it, or the history of its development the thing itself. Yet we often accept one of these as the phenomenon. When we do we have taken the target phenomenon as less than it is in its original human context. Our investigation, our approach to the phenomenon, is unsatisfying in the sense that it remains, in L. Farber's term, "phenomenally thin" (1966). Its human qualities, its experiential qualities, have been lost.

When we do not approach the phenomenon as such, but instead

substitute an operation or explanation of it, we have never closed the gap between our research and the phenomenon as we live it. There can be a common starting point, a common definition or operation, without ever touching the phenomenon which we intended to study. Again, introversion is a case in point. It has remained elusive even to those investigators who do not doubt the fact of its existence. However, this "loss" of the phenomenon is not peculiar to the problem of introversion but is a hazard born more generally of our present methods in psychology.

An alternative way of proceeding would be to carry continual concern about losing the phenomenon as experienced. The goals in this approach might be, first, to locate the target phenomenon in experience, and second, to describe it with an eye to what it requires to be this and no other phenomenon. By what method can we indulge this concern and achieve these goals? Is there a method which is at base experiential which could utilize the results of traditional objective methods? We desire an experiential method which does not treat objective methods or their results simply or exclusively by walling itself off from them. As sensitive as we are to the problem of "losing" the phenomenon, we nevertheless espouse an experiential method which gains its ends through a constructive integration with objective methods.

All of these goals, except the latter, find expression in a school of psychology called "phenomenological psychology." Phenomenology originated in philosophy as a call to return to the thing itself as experienced. The philosophical approach is an attempt to bracket or suspend all that which is not the thing itself. What remains is a description of the essential or constitutive qualities of the phenomenon, its thingness, as it were.

In the sections to follow we shall first outline the general approach of phenomenological psychology and some of its substantive results. Phenomenological psychology will be distinguished from positivism both as a method and as a view of man. These sections are intended to serve as an introduction to phenomenology for those unfamiliar with it. They should serve to facilitate a reading of the descriptive formulation of introversion and to point to further material from which a deeper understanding of phenomenology may be gained. After indicating the extent of the differences between positivism and phenomenology we shall turn about by suggesting how they may be integrated as a working method.

Phenomenology: The General Approach

Phenomenology as it has been transplanted from philosophy to psychology* and as it since has developed within psychology is an "attempt to clarify what is essential in naive experience" (Van Kaam, 1966, p. 142). This effort is explicitly counter to an exclusively positivistic or objectivistic approach. The phenomenological psychologist would have investigators "remain with what they immediately perceive and not get lost in 'scientific' abstractions, derivations, explanations, and calculations . . ." (Boss, 1963, p. 30). Or, in the same vein, they would have us "linger with them [the phenomena as they are presented to us] sufficiently long to become fully aware of what they tell us directly about their meaning and essence" (Boss, 1963, p. 30).

Much of phenomenological philosophy, as distinct from phenomenological psychology, is devoted to a rigorous and exhaustive exposition of the essentials of experience and of the method by which one arrives at them.† By essentials of experience we mean such things as its structure, its essential components and how they are related to each other, its modes of appearing, the "constitution" of phenomena in experience (the steps by which they emerge or are crystallized), and the like (Spiegelberg, 1969, 2: 659).

Phenomenological psychologists utilize only some aspects of both the method and the findings of these philosophical inquiries; and these they have adapted in the borrowing. For example, a notion central to Husserl's method is that of the "reduction." This technical

*We have relied primarily on the following writers loosely divided into those in philosophy and then those in psychology. We list them in order of increasing difficulty of presentation in the hope that the interested reader will find this sequence a productive one for further exploration. The order in no way reflects the importance of their particular contribution to phenomenology.

Spiegelberg, 1969; Sadler, 1969; Natanson, 1970; Luijpen, 1969; Buber, 1955, 1958; Kockelmans, 1967; Sartre, 1966; Koestenbaum, in Husserl, 1970b; Farber, 1967; Merleau-Ponty, 1962, 1963; Husserl, 1970a, 1970b; Heidegger, 1970.

Van den Berg, 1955, 1961; Straus, 1966; Boss, 1963; Buytendijk, in Ruitenbeek, 1962; Binswanger, in May, 1967; Van Kaam, 1966; Gendlin, 1962; Sonneman, 1954.

†Husserl in his writings is additionally concerned with attaining an "absolutely valid knowledge of things" (Kockelmans, 1967, p. 26). A phenomenological philosophy in his view has "the aim of grounding science absolutely" (Husserl, 1970a, p. 8). It seeks to describe the grounds of knowing, what makes knowing possible. By returning to experience as-given and as-constituted a fulcrum might be established. This fulcrum would be a point of absolute certainty upon which all science could be built. Phenomenologists since Husserl have been more concerned with employing the phenomenological method in the service of describing an ontology, a science of existence or being (Heidegger, Sartre, and, to a lesser extent, Merleau-Ponty).

term is not to be confused with the "reductionism," mentioned above, to which an objectivistic approach is prone. Husserl does not use this term to mean "making less than," since he was critical of the Occam's razor principle of economizing or simplifying which he saw operative in positivistic science (Spiegelberg, 1969, 2: 657). The term rather refers more literally to a "leading back" (Spiegelberg, 1969, 1: 133). Through the general procedure of reduction, an attitude in which one can "perceive things as they are in themselves, independently of any prejudice" is achieved (Kockelmans, 1967, p. 30). It is an attempt to leave aside or bracket off sequentially all beliefs, theories, or presuppositions about the world, the other person, and the self. The phenomenological method according to Husserl largely proceeds through a series of these reductions. They are divided generally as follows: The eidetic reduction (from facts to essences) and the phenomenological reduction which itself includes the "bracketing of being," the reduction of the cultural world to the world of immediate experience, and the transcendental reduction (Kockelmans, 1967, p. 31).

Phenomenological psychology roughly follows Husserl in only two of these reductions. First, it brackets being; it "forgets" for the moment the question of the "reality" of objects. It attempts to follow things as they appear in experience without judgment as to their existence. Second, as we suggested earlier, these investigators, in their effort to reach the essential characteristics of an experience, expend considerable effort to bracket off cultural influences, habits of thought, and perhaps most important, theoretical biases of the most implicit and embedded kind.

In a way this idea that there are factors or contaminants which can block us from an understanding of a particular phenomenon is familiar to us in psychology. One thinks of the emphasis on recognizing experimenter bias, "demand characteristics," and other artifactual but assumedly controllable factors or contaminants inherent in experimental settings. More generally, however, and more subtly, the idea runs counter to some of the assumptions in the approach of the traditional experimental psychologist. We can imagine a proponent of this latter approach responding: But those things, language habit, thought habit, cultural and social influence and the like, which you call contaminants are not that at all. They are the determinants of the phenomenon in experience. (He would probably say the determinants of the behavior.) They determine it in its form, in its particulars, and in its expression. He would maintain that we cannot study the phenomenon without taking these contaminants into account through varying them and mapping out their contribution and effect on the phenomenon. In fact, he would maintain that this mapping out of the effect of the contaminants on the phenomenon and their relation to the phenomenon are the study of the phenomenon. More radically, his assumption is that the mapping and relation taken together constitute the phenomenon. The causal and correlative nexus is the phenomenon. The contaminants, the aspects to be bracketed for the phenomenologist, are for him very much the phenomenon. To use a simple example, if the phenomenon of interest is greed, what the greedy person hoards, under what conditions, other characteristics of the greedy person, and how he came to be greedy, are inseparable from and, indeed, are the study of greed.

Phenomenology, on the other hand, contends that there are characteristics of a phenomenon which cut across and are prior to culture, language, setting, and the abstractions encrusted in them; and that these characteristics are constitutive of the phenomenon. Part of what is constitutive of greed is a "filling of space" (Binswanger in Sadler, 1969, p. 133). Through bracketing such considerations as the particulars of culture and setting, which might determine what is filled with what; the possible genesis of greed; theories as to the "dynamics" of greed; and the like we return to and see directly this "filling" aspect and other requisite aspects.

This general introduction to a phenomenological approach brings to mind a demand we made of Jung in chapter 1. We were critical of his failure to describe the introverted attitude before it wends its particularizing way through various interactions with culture, psychological function, degree of neuroticism, and the like. We were also critical of his tendency to conceal the phenomenon behind theories and metaphors, and to confuse these theories with the phenomenon. Further, we noted that he employed theories whose assumptions prejudice the description of a phenomenon as experienced. What we were essentially doing was pointing out that his work might have been greatly enhanced by increased attention to a phenomenological method.

Phenomenological psychology generally stops on the descriptive level. It does so not because it sees itself serving only a propaedeutic function in a larger scientific enterprise, but because the whole logic of phenomenology as a way to proceed points to a description of the constitutive characteristics of a phenomenon as the proper goal of an investigation. Such a description is the closest approach to the thing itself save for experiencing it oneself. A description is, or can be, phenomenally thick.

One of the basic conclusions of Husserl's philosophy is that the person, the scientist included, never perceives an object except with reference to himself. There is no possibility of a "naive naturalism," of perceiving or of studying something out there as it is, independent of us. The view that "there is an external, 'real' world, existing in itself, independent of man" is itself a presupposition, one which is the general working principle of the natural sciences (Boss, 1963, p. 75). For the phenomenologist, however, our relation to the world is such that reality is necessarily perspectival (Merleau-Ponty, 1963, p. 186). Reality as we originally know it consists always in a particular view of a thing. To return to the thing itself our program cannot be to eliminate the "observer," the experiencing being, but rather must be to move back to him, to take as reality an embodied view of a thing.

The phenomenological psychologist as investigator, then, does not assume himself an observer of a phenomenon thought of as external to him. His stance involves his always being in the thick of it. The phenomenon is not something which can be kept at a distance and reflected on from some vantage point idealized as neutral. He does not even employ the strategy that his peculiar experience of the phenomenon is a "bias," which although inherent in observation may be "controlled." Rather, he brackets or suspends this traditional naturalistic premise. This bracketing of the possibility of studying the phenomenon from outside of it, carrying as it does a conceptual baggage which places a barrier between the experiencer and the experienced, leaves him free to have the phenomenon directly. As Van den Berg graphically but tellingly describes, the investigator's solution is to become the phenomenon, to let it take him over. "To write a treatise on swimming, he will first go for a swim" (1955, p. 62). Only then can he begin to locate its essential characteristics.

This approach has some apparent similarity to that of the classical introspectionist. However, the latter's method is more closely related to that of the laboratory experimentalist.* He differs from

---

*"Introspective psychology detected, on the perimeter of the physical world, a zone of consciousness in which physical concepts are no longer valid, but the psychologist still believed consciousness to be no more than a sector of being, and he decided to explore this sector as the physicist explores his" (Merleau-Ponty, 1962, p. 59).

the experimentalist only in the size of his sample with his "N" of one; and in the fact that the experimentalist and the subject are the same person. There is the same effort to create or reproduce experimentally the phenomenon in a location that is said to be external to a neutral observer who then measures its effects. Both the introspectionist and the experimental psychologist attempt to recreate the phenomenon either in the lab or in the part of self where they can observe it while keeping themselves or at least their reflective selves at some remove from it.

In contrast, the phenomenological psychologist attempts to let the phenomenon speak directly to him by engaging himself in it. The necessity of directly experiencing the phenomenon as a first step in proceeding will become clearer as we turn to some of the constitutive features of experience set forth by phenomenology. After presenting them, we shall return to a closer description of an integrated phenomenological approach.

Lived Experience

Givenness of lived experience

Phenomenological psychology is primarily concerned with naive experience. One defining characteristic of naive experience is that it is given. Say we are experiencing something at a particular moment. Before we reflect on it, before we say to ourselves what it is we are having in the moment, it is there for us. It is immediately there for us, prereflectively, preconceptually, tacitly. It is immanently disclosed to us. It is given, then, in the sense of already there for us. This givenness is most striking in such moments as when we are reading an interesting book or having a heated discussion. In these moments we are engaged or absorbed. When there is this absorption of self or forgetting of self in the moment or in the participation in the moment, the givenness, the lived moment's quality of immanence is clearest.

That things are directly disclosed to us in lived experience is evident also in another dramatic example. Recall that moment in which the telephone rings and we respond to it with general arousal and even with movement toward it, before we say to ourselves "the phone is ringing." Or, again, recall how sometimes the first ring already grips the heart before we become "aware" that it is that long awaited call. Lived experience has this bodily aspect. It is always touching us and is immediately concretely felt or embodied.

The lived moment is distinguished by some writers from "reflective" (Van den Berg, 1955, p. 61) or reflected or postconceptual experience. Reflected experience involves an objectifying of lived experience (Van Kaam, 1966, p. 33). It is disengaged while lived experience is engaged. This objectifying is antithetical to the lived experience of the moment. "If we reflect on the moment, it becomes an *article* of knowledge" (Farber, 1966, p. 136, emphasis ours). The lived experience in its givenness and its engagement or absorption of the person precludes his making of it an article or an object. Immanence and reflectivity are more or less distinct modes of experience. Incidentally, the distinction here is not at all the Jungian one between thinking and feeling. Intellectual discussion or the activity of reading a book, both "thinking" tasks, may be experienced through a being absorbed in the moment. Conversely, the predominant mode by which a person reflects on something may be through the "feeling function."

Lived experience and its constitutive features of givenness and absorption are not part of a conceptual frame. Lived experience is the primary material of phenomenology. Its features are descriptive findings as to "how it is" in lived experience. The logic of the phenomenological approach demands that qualities like givenness not be treated like slices of a pie divided according to the dictates of a particular framework. "Givenness" has a particular and precise experiential referent.

It is a central task of phenomenology to make lived experience explicit through a description of it. One particular difficulty in accomplishing this task involves the present constitutive feature of lived experience. If our only "framework" is the expressed purpose of describing experience as it appears, and if it is given, we cannot bring to it. If it is given, to receive it we must approach it unarmed by particular categories of thought. Again, to describe the experience of swimming, we must swim. But then what? Having experienced it in the moment, how do we arrive at an understanding of it on an explicit and reflective level? When we reflect on it, when we make of it an object, do we not rob it of one of its essential features, its self-absorbing immanence? And then have we not lost it? We shall return to this question at a later point.

It should be clear that lived experience does not refer to a peculiar or occasional subset of experiences within a much larger round of ordinary everyday experiencing. It is not a realm composed of discrete moments narrow in range and isolated from the rest of experience like the sudden "discovery" of a previously "unconscious" tapping of one's foot in time to the music, or the striking sense of closeness given in a heavy autumn dusk, or the "getting lost in" lives depicted on the movie screen. It is rather the continuous way in which we experience the world and ourselves in it. It is what we are having at every moment before we say what it is we are having. There is always available a particular bodily-sense, a felt-experience at every moment. As such, it is central to human existence.

Further, lived experience is itself a way of knowing the world, a way which is other than objectifying it. It is a knowing that is at the moment of knowing preobjective, prereflective, and bodily felt. Not only is it a central part of human existence, it is itself a way of knowing more about that existence. For these reasons and others it is held in high regard by phenomenologists. Some writers maintain further that lived experience is the ground of all reflected experience, i.e., that every objectification has its basis in a given preconceptual experiencing (Van Kaam, 1966); or that lived experience is a necessary and intimate part of the structure of all reflected experience (Polanyi, 1966); or at least that the interaction between it and reflected experience is what "creates" and advances meaning for the person (Gendlin, 1962).

In-the-world character of lived experience

As we have noted, Husserl asserts that we cannot describe the world without reference to the self that is describing it. In its later development, phenomenology adds constitutive features of experience which yield the inverse of this assertion: We cannot describe a person without describing the world which he inhabits.

In describing the in-the-world character of lived experience, which clarifies in what sense we always "inhabit" the world, phenomenologists often begin with a refutation of a metaphysic identified with Descartes. It is the operation of the Cartesian dualism as an assumptive base, they contend, which has rendered our attempts to understand the nature of experience ineffective and unsatisfactory. It is the pervasiveness of Cartesian thinking, indeed, that necessitates a phenomenology.

A brief presentation of this philosophy will set the background for phenomenology's critique of it and lead naturally to the present constitutive feature of experience. Descartes defined man as consisting of two separate and distinct substances, mind and body. Both mind and body, he asserted, are things. They are simply opposite kinds of things. One occupies space and has weight and one does not. Man as mind is a thinking thing, a *res cogitans.* This thinking thing is somehow housed in the body. As such it is cut off from the body and, more importantly, it is cut off by the body from the world. Mind is internal and private, and body is external and public. In his later writings Descartes, while retaining this dualistic view, connected its two parts through a mechanistic linkage. The body is a machine governed by a second machine, mind, which is somehow internal to it, although it occupies no space and has no weight. He suggested that physical stimuli must cross over from body into mind and then out again. He hypothesized the pineal gland as this point of connection between the two otherwise separated things.*

Almost all psychological theories assume this dualism of the mind and body. Concomitantly they tend to define the "person" independent of the world in which he lives, consciousness outside of the object of consciousness, and subjectivity without reference to objectivity. The Cartesian metaphysic limits or establishes the way in which we conceive of the self/world relation. Guided by this implicit dualistic presupposition theories generally reflect major concern with one of its poles to the relative exclusion of the other. There are idealistic and empirical theories (Van Kaam, 1966, p. 202), intrapsychic and environmental or behavioristic theories, subjective and objective theories. Common to one pole of these dichotomies is the doctrine of the "worldless subject" (Van den Berg in Ruitenbeek, 1962, p. 103). This "myth of the encapsulated ego," as it is called by critics of the Cartesian dualism (A. Watts, 1963, p. 18), is the most striking instance of the person or subject removed from the world. He is trapped in his skin. "We are demarcated from the world by this envelope of skin" (Bleibtreu, 1968, p. 63). Complementing this conception and matching it in experiential thinness is the doctrine of the subjectless world common to theories representing the other pole. In these theories, often referred to as "empty box" theories, there is in effect no person. There is only the world as a set of

*It requires little stretch of mind to recognize in this mechanically joined world/body-mind-body/world sequence the S-O-R frame of much of behaviorism.

stimuli, the sensory organism, and the motor response. Both sets of theories require fairly elaborate conceptual bridges in order to put the person back into the world.

The task should begin with the consideration of the person as a being in-the-world, where he always has been. For Descartes, consciousness consists of intransitive statements of the form "I think," "I imagine."* They constitute subjectivity and are the only psychological reality. This reality is distinct from and external to the reality of the world.

Brentano takes the first step away from this position with his modification of Descartes' "I think" to "I think of (an object)." Consciousness is consciousness of something. It is never the Cartesian "a thinking," "a perceiving." It is always a thinking of a tree, a perceiving of a house. Consciousness is a pointing, a directedness. It is always beyond itself. It is a pointing-to-something-that-is-not-itself. This characteristic of consciousness of always tending toward or intending an object is called "intentionality."

For our purposes, Husserl completes the emigration of the subject with his broadening of Brentano's notion of intentionality. For Brentano consciousness has a quality of directedness. It is no longer exclusively concerned with and restricted to itself, a thing thinking. However, for Brentano there is still a rift between the objective world and the world-as-experienced, the world of our consciousness. His thinking about experience implies, as did Descartes', two realities. While consciousness is not occupied with some inner world or self, the object to which it points is not the external object. It is, schematically, in parentheses. Consciousness though intentional never reaches the object in the world. It deals only with an image or representation of it. The person remains, for Brentano, separated from the world, although always oriented toward it.

Husserl argues that there is only one reality. The actual object is the object of intentional consciousness. For example, when we perceive this house, we do not experience an image of it; we experience the house itself. Experience is not simply a pointing from where it is to out beyond itself. It is not a thing which is directed, at the periphery of its own sphere or reality (a subjective or internal reality), to a second sphere which it does not touch (an objective or external reality). It is rather always outside itself. It is in-the-world.

*The following schematic mode of presentation of material on Descartes, Brentano, and Husserl is borrowed from Van den Berg (in Ruitenbeek, 1962).

Another way to describe this is to think of experience as a "radical openness" onto the world (Van Kaam, 1966, p. 8). Again, this does not mean that experience is something in itself and open to something else. Experience is itself an opening. Its embeddedness in the world ensures that we do not see an image of the world on a screen that is not the world. We see the world itself because experience is in-the-world.

In addition to this present sense of intentionality, of experience inseparable from the world it intends, Husserl also includes under this term experience-as-constituted. Constituting intentionality refers to the fact that "the object of my consciousness . . . is something meant, constructed, projected, constituted, in short, *intended* by me" (Koestenbaum in Husserl, 1970b, p. xxvii; his emphasis). With its directedness to that which it is not, consciousness or experiencing is always immediately answering the question: What do you intend, what do you mean, or what is meant? Intentionality refers to experience's meaning-giving feature. (As we have noted earlier, meaning in lived experience is tacit, only felt, not yet in words.) Intending is an act that gives objects meaning, that, in this sense, constitutes or builds up objects. Experiencing is a continual building and rebuilding of the world. An intentional analysis of lived experience, then, also involves a constitutive analysis, an analysis of how meaning is constituted through or in experience (Kockelmans, 1967, p. 35). Incidentally, there is an apparent contradiction between this essential characteristic of lived experience and its quality of givenness described earlier. How can it both be already there, given to me in the moment, and at the same, built up by me, given meaning by me? We shall discuss these and other analogous antinomies when we return to the problem of introversion below. In this antinomous structure we shall find a ground for the I/E difference.

A final approach to the in-the-world character of lived experience is to draw attention to the relational nature of experience. Here we move briefly and of necessity to ontological considerations, and to the work of Heidegger (1970) and an existential analyst who followed him in much of his thinking, Medard Boss (1963).

Both the present feature of lived experience and one discussed earlier, its givenness, suggest that there is a very profound relation between the person and the world, one which is given in the moment. The intimacy of this relation defines or constitutes the person experientially.

What is meant by the relational nature of lived experience is approached by the notion of "physiognomic" or dynamic perception as described by Werner (in Baldwin, 1968), Schachtel (1966), Straus (1966), and others. A physiognomic perception is the immediately given "attitude" of the object. The object or scene or situation is experienced as menacing, huge, welcoming, small, and so on. For example, some people perceive in a ∪-shaped form on card 7 of the Rorschach, the attitude of opening or vulnerability, others perceive it as a protective harbor (Schachtel, 1966, pp. 123ff). Here the experience is relational in the limited sense that it has an immediately given meaning according to its perceived relation to the viewer. It is bigger or smaller than him; and he is smaller or bigger than it.

The relational nature of the lived moment is akin to this physiognomic quality of perception, but it refers to a quality of experience in which any remaining sense of the subject/object split is eliminated. In lived experience, since we do not objectify, since we do not experience things as objects distinct from self as observer, there is no separation between self or subject and object. The opposite of separation is relation or relatedness (Buber, 1958, p. 23). "In the beginning [prior to reflection] is relation" (Buber, p. 18). There are not two entities, the subject or person or observer and the object, thing observed, or world. In lived experience, there is one entity formed of the meeting of the two, consisting in the relation between the two. There is only the subject/object encounter.

When, for example, we perceive or think of this house, when we become engaged in it, there is not ourselves and the house. We are not in our heads while the object is out there. It is not accurate, either, to say we are a pointing toward the object. "During the being absorbed in thinking of the house there before me, there is nothing to be found of an I that thinks, nor of an of, to which the thinking would be directed" (Van den Berg in Ruitenbeek, 1962, p. 103). The answer to the question where are we? or where is the person? is in-the-world or in a relation to the world. What the person is, is a being-in-the-world. This "location" of the self outside of any circumscribed or internal sphere; this coming out from or standing out from (*ekstasis*, Boss, 1963, p. 43) and meeting of another object or person wherein is formed a "new" psychological reality is what is referred to as being-in-the-world. In lived experience we do not simply give a significance to objects, nor do we only perceive an attitude in them vis-à-vis ourself; we encounter them. Our experience of self is not of a relation between us and the object, but rather consists in a relation with it. A person's involvement in the world is so complete as to constitute what there is of him. We are absorbed in the encounter and we are the encounter.

In other terms, what there is of the person, what the person is, is a "being there" (*dasein*, Boss, 1963, p. 39). He has his being over there at the house. There is no self, no I here seeing the house there. The existence that is the person, as distinguished from all other kinds of beings, is a being-there. Being there refers to the fundamental relation of person and world, his being threaded to it (Merleau-Ponty, 1962, p. xiii)—the fact of his being-in-the-world. The particular relation that is the person in a given moment is a description of his particular mode of being-in-the-world. It is a description of how he is in the moment. It answers the question: How is he being-there?

Finally, and again to suggest the apparent contradictory nature of experience, experience is world-disclosing. We "luminate" the house; we disclose it and we build it up (Boss, 1963, p. 37). Yet at the same time that we disclose it, we are in that moment the world we disclose. A person is a world-disclosing being.

We quote Boss here more fully to review a number of the points in this section:

> Actually man is not merely *involved* in his relationships toward a particular being of his world, he does not merely *have* such a relationship among his other properties or abilities. He *is* at any given moment nothing but *in* and *as* this or that perceiving, instinctual, impulsive, emotional, imaginative, dreaming, thinking, acting, willing, or wishing relationship toward the things which he encounters. In other words, man always and from the beginning fulfills his existence *in* and *as* one or the other mode of behavior in regard to something or somebody. In this sense, man is fundamentally "out in the world" and *with* the things he encounters. His existence is originally a "being-in-the-world. ..." [Boss, 1963, pp. 33–34; his emphasis]

With this brief survey of some structures of experience according to phenomenology, it should be clearer: (1) that to describe a person (including, of course, an introvert), we must describe his world-as-experienced; and (2) how phenomenology necessarily launches itself out of a traditional Cartesian dualistic conception of things.

An Integrated Phenomenological Approach

The relation between lived and reflected experience

We return again to the problem of making lived experience explicit through a description of it. We have already indicated how psychological investigation has typically excluded the experiential nature of phenomena. A positivistic psychology objectifies the phenomenon and in so doing thins it, hollows it, loses it as-experienced. Further, it takes this objectification as the thing itself, building a world which is the composite of nexuses between the objectification and others of similar character and origin. The resultant world is emptied of the world in which we are always embedded. What is confusedly called the "real" world is actually an idealized one. This abstract world, separated from and unencumbered by the world-as-lived, requires a philosophical base such as the Cartesian dualism upon which to stand.

We have described how we can circumvent this idealized world of our conceptions and return to lived experience by approaching it unarmed, by simply "having" it, by participating in the moment. This initial stance to the phenomenon, allowing a return to it, involves an "inhabiting" (Merleau-Ponty), an "indwelling" (Buber), or an "entering into" it (Van den Berg). But because of the character of lived experience the return is momentary and the moment itself is elusive. We can return to it but we cannot hold on to it or pin it down. It is always only a tacit knowing and we need to make it explicit. Our having of it is inseparable from our embeddedness in it, and yet we need to step out of it to record it. This is the dilemma. It is ". . . like seizing a spinning top to catch its motion" (James, 1961, p. 28). In Merleau-Ponty's terms, lived experience or "existence" has a thickness and an opacity such that "as thinking subject we are never the unreflected subject that we seek to know" (1962, p. 62).

Clearly, to describe a phenomenon as experienced we require a more elaborate and considered investigatory stance. It must not only allow us to enter readily into our experiencing, but, as well, to emerge with it intact. To define this stance a number of questions must first be addressed: What in general is the relation between lived experience and subsequent reflected experience? More specifically, what is the relation between the thing as-experienced and an eventual description of that experiencing? In what sense may that description be said to be valid and what is the criterion for its validity? Further, in the other direction, what is the relationship between our reflection on a particular phenomenon and subsequent engagement in that phenomenon? Finally, does this relationship allow us to integrate the results of objective methods in this study of lived experience?

Eugene Gendlin deals with these questions systematically and practically in a fruitful way (1962). His description of lived experi-

ence, which he refers to as "experiencing," emphasizes its embeddedness, and stresses how it always refers to what is going on in
situations or "how we are" in a situation. Experiencing is a sense of
what is going on at every moment that is felt but not yet in words.
Gendlin calls this sense of the situation we are in, the "felt-meaning"
of experiencing. Experiencing as felt-meaning is embodied. It is given
as a bodily sense. Here are some examples he offers illustrating these
points:

When someone is about to jump at you, you feel it in your "gut." When
someone is in a complicated way going to hurt, again you feel it in your gut. Just
as a golfer feels in his body, in the position of his feet, and in the muscular sense
of his swing, the whole scene in front of him, so do we bodily experience the
complexity of our situations and interactions. [1969, p. 8]

Another example of how experiencing is felt-meaning sensed on a
"concrete bodily level" often occurs when we participate in a discussion. Just prior to speaking, perhaps while we wait to get the present
speaker's eye, we already "have" what we shall say or try to express
(Gendlin, p. 131). Our sense of it is already lodged with us in a
concrete bodily way. We "know" our point although we do not yet
have it in words. We are experiencing it in a "bodily way" only. More
generally "experiencing," in that it is felt-meaning and in that it has
or is a bodily expression, is a preconceptual undifferentiated mass of
many aspects that are bodily felt. The concrete bodily sense is of the
whole situation we are in. It is the felt-mass of all its many aspects. It
is a "pre-conceptual richness" (1969, p. 7).

There are at least two gains here in Gendlin's description of lived
experience or "experiencing." The emphasis on experiencing as concrete bodily feeling obliterates the mind/body dualism. In the same
vein an immediately present bodily sense of a situation undercuts
any self/world dichotomy while underscoring the ontological truth
that a person is a being-in-the-world. Second, and more important for
our present purposes, Gendlin's emphasis on meaning as only felt in
lived experience allows us to examine the relationship between
felt-meaning and reflected or conceptual meaning.

Gendlin begins to describe this relation with the assertion that we
can refer directly to an implicit felt-meaning (pp. 91–100, 1962). We
can point to it, mark it off or set it off, find it. For example, we see a
painting and have a particular response to it. We can refer to that
complex of felt-meaning before we can formulate it in words. We can
refer to "my feeling about it" and by so doing we can focus our

attention on that bodily felt-mass. Similarly, we can refer to "what I wanted to say," "all that about how I get along with my wife," and, in general, how I am in a given situation.

Giving attention to or "focusing" on a felt-meaning through "direct reference" is not reentry into the lived moment or the set of lived moments in which such a bodily sensed meaning occurred. It is a reference to the stuff of a moment as-experienced. Through direct reference we point to what we were having in a moment without engaging ourselves in it, without again forgetting ourselves in the moment. This pointing, then, is access to a lived moment, to a felt-meaning. It is an access that is independent of the particular felt-meaning in that it does not change it. It does not include reentering it and furthering it. Whatever minimal explicit meaning the pointer might have ("that," "all of that"), the particular felt-meaning functions independently of that meaning. On the other hand, direct reference is not an empty pointing, as one might designate a room with no sense of what is in it. It is a pointing which actually reaches to the felt bodily-sense of a moment. It touches and delimits a particular concrete bodily-sense. When we say, "what I wanted to say was . . ." before we complete the statement we already can be pointing to the felt-meaning, it can already be experientially available to us.

This may not seem like much, but really it is a significant breakthrough. The notion of direct reference to "experiencing" strikes to the heart of the lived/reflected experience dilemma. With this as a starting point, Gendlin can then work out how we can approach and capture lived experience without destroying it. A particular lived experience, with this independent access to it through direct reference, can be the subject of our discussion and of our investigation. Gendlin applies this initial notion of experiencing to the problem of therapeutic change (1969). The therapist can instruct and actively guide his client back to his problem as-experienced, before rationalizations and intellectualizations disguise it and bury it.

With direct reference as a starting point, while we are not at the same time in the moment and reflecting on it, we are pointing to what we were having of the moment in its totality as it was tacitly experienced. We can refer to a lived moment without the presuppositions of any reflected conceptual frame. We can objectify it, make it the object of our attention without tampering with it, reducing it, or the like. Certainly, this is as close as we might hope to get to seizing the spinning top without disrupting its movement.

Still, with this access, how do we describe a particular felt-meaning? We can refer directly to it, but how do we "have" it in words? What is the relationship between it and our explicit meanings, our reflected thoughts?

Following Gendlin, then, let us say that at any given moment we are having a felt-meaning. As we focus our attention on it, words can come from it. Felt-meaning, when we focus on it, can have a selective function (p. 107, 1962). It can select symbols that conceptualize, express, formulate, or in general "explicate" it.* Before speaking, words "come to us," "symbols present themselves" (p. 107, 1962). When we focus, or when we refer directly to a particular felt-meaning, we suddenly have an explicit thought.

This is helpful, but we require the converse, too. "Explication" and direct reference operate only with respect to a felt-meaning that is already present at that moment. We need a way to locate any felt-meaning that interests us so that we can refer to it and eventually explicate it. If we are to investigate a particular aspect of experiencing, a particular problem, we must have access to it at our own command and when it suits us.

There is another relationship between explicit "meaning" or symbols and felt-meaning that provides just this requisite converse of explication. Symbols, in the form of an initial formulation or description, can "call forth" a particular felt-meaning. A "formulation" of a phenomenon can function to "lift out" that phenomenon as concretely felt. Gendlin refers to this relation as "recognition" (pp. 100–106, 1962). Recognition and direct reference are similar in that they, unlike explication, both move toward a felt-meaning. However, the "that" of direct reference only points. It is dependent on the immediate presence of the felt-meaning. The "formulation" when it functions to "recognize" is independent of felt-meaning in that it can call it up. It has the power of a particular felt-meaning that Aladdin has over his own genie. Further, while the "that" of direct reference "means" only in that it points, a formulation "means" in the sense of representing or conceptualizing. For example, the symbolization, "the kind of anger I feel in a situation where I . . .," represents a particular felt-meaning as it lifts it out.

*Our earlier usage of the term "explication," particularly in chapter 1, was not in the specific sense of Gendlin's term.

In that it symbolizes rather than only points, however, there is a dependence in the other direction. The symbols of the formulation "mean" what they conceptualize, but what they conceptualize is the particular felt-meaning (p. 102, 1962). The symbolization does not have meaning unless it calls forth a felt-meaning. The relation between a formulation that means and felt-meaning is such that the latter is the experienced meaning of the former. The felt-meaning *"constitutes our having of the meaning"* (pp. 101–102, 1962, Gendlin's emphasis). Not only must we feel the explicit symbols on a concrete bodily level for them to mean, but also that bodily feeling is the experience of that meaning. This last is an important point which is undoubtedly familiar (tacitly felt) but one which is generally not stated as such (explicated). A formulation, an explicit thought, "means" only to the extent that it has a recognition function. The felt-meaning that it calls forth is the experience of the meaning of the formulation.

A symbolization, then, through recognition calls up a felt-meaning, as it must if it is to mean anything. Further, we can employ it to call up a specific felt-meaning of interest. There is another way in which the felt-meaning is not the servant of the formulation. After it lifts out a phenomenon which we can then sense concretely, there is what Gendlin calls a "response." The "response" is a kind of comparison between the formulation and the then noticed phenomenon. We can say, "yes, that's it" or we can say, "that's what I was getting at, but I'm not quite saying it right." The response is an immediately given acceptance or rejection of the formulation. Note, however, that if we reject it, we still have the phenomenon to which it led us. Once a formulation has led us to a felt-meaning we can have independent access to it. We can directly refer to it. We then can modify our formulation of it through explication until we obtain a positive response, a "that's it." This "response" is an experiential criterion which operates in both the process of recognition and that of explication. We can always consider symbolization with reference to a particular felt-meaning and say, "that's not quite what I mean" (p. 109, 1962). There is this check available which we utilize automatically in everyday life as we move back and forth between felt-meaning and reflection. We shall return to its description below when we examine further the problem of validity.

It is clear from all of this that felt-meaning, although a particular bodily-felt experiencing, requires a formulation to "mean," it must be explicated; and conversely, a symbolization must lift out (lead to the recognition of) a felt-meaning before it means. In fact, "meaning" is precisely a particular relation between experiencing and symbolization: a pointing to the first by the second (recognition), or a selecting of the second by the first (explication).

What has been described thus far about the relationship between lived experience and reflected experience, including the experiential check, leaves open the possibility that the words which eventually symbolize a felt-meaning are in the felt-meaning ready to be set free. This is not the case. Felt-meanings do not contain thoughts or concepts as a bag might contain marbles neatly labelled with titles or terms. "Experiencing" or lived experience is not a phenomenon composed of different thoughts in the company of respective "affects," as in the psychoanalytic notion of the contents of the "unconscious." The undifferentiated mass that is a felt-meaning does not itself become explicit. It can yield the explicit and conversely the explicit can "locate" it in the ways we have described, following Gendlin. Felt-meaning and symbolization have particular connections to each other, affect each other in consistent, specifiable ways, but they remain radically distinct phenomena, different kinds of "thing."

Experiencing is not like becoming aware of a bag of labelled marbles, nor is it even similar to a marble or a bag of marbles or any other "thing." It does not consist of concepts as does a formulation, even one of its own formulations, nor is it a "thing" with the class of properties associated with such.* We think of things as having pieces, parts, or units. Experiencing, however, is not a set of units of anything. Our formulation of it does not have or use up or uncover increasingly large segments of it. A formulation is not related to felt-meaning in degree of comprehensiveness. Since it has no units felt-meaning is "non-numerical" (p. 152, 1962). It does not consist in a determinate number of experiences. It follows that our specification or symbolization of it can be composed of any number of explicit statements. A "response" of "that's it" can come with one phrase or with a highly differentiated description. Finally, along this line, "experiencing" is not itself organized in schematic relationships. In "experiencing," experiences are not related to each other. For example, experiences, in "experiencing," or as we experience them, are not "close" to each other or otherwise related to each other except as symbolization makes it so (p. 153, 1962). Symbolization

---

*Technically, it would not be accurate, then, to refer to *a* felt-meaning although in this informal presentation we have not kept to this.

makes or creates the schematic relations. Relations between different experiences exist only in and through their formulations. Further, consistent with the nonunitary nature of experiencing, a number of different schemes can specify a felt-meaning. The "to-be-specified experiences are capable of being specified according to many schemes" (p. 154, 1962).

Experiencing or lived experience is always unspecified and unsymbolized, always only felt. It is always "not fully determined," ununified and unschematic. Perhaps it is now clearer that our formulations of experiencing cannot be simply a locating or identifying of meanings waiting there to be disclosed or clarified like so many momentarily opaque marbles. Our symbolization is a creating of meaning in the sense that our formulations work on felt-meaning, bringing out of its lack of unity, number, and schema, its lack of "thingness," new entities which diminish these lacks. Our formulation creates a thing out of what is and what remains only a felt undifferentiated mass.

But now we are in danger of losing what we have gained from earlier discussion. We are making the relationship between experiencing and formulation appear too loose, too indeterminate, as if anything goes. The formulation, although it is a creative act, does not unitize and schematize *ex nihilo*. It cannot indulge its own artful whim and remain meaningful. Again, meaning is a particular relation between experiencing or felt-meaning and its explicit description. Felt-meaning as we experience it does not have set units, but neither is it a completely formless lump which stands motionless unaffecting or in turn unaffected by our formulation. The relation between the two is really a strict one with its own rules. If we adhere to them, the validity of our formulations can be assured.

As we have described, we have a check: we can tell whether or not we have found words for a lived experience and, conversely, whether an initially disembodied intellectualization has been embodied. There is a response of "that's it" or "no, not quite." Words that really "come from" felt-meaning have what Gendlin describes as a "felt-relief, a felt-shift" (p. 5, 1969). For example, when a patient finally puts in words what he has been afraid of he may visibly sigh with relief, " 'Yeah, that's what it is, all right' " (p. 5, 1969). This felt-release is followed by the movement of the felt-meaning, which provides the basis for a second kind of check on our formulations of any phenomenon as-experienced.

The felt-meaning does not stand still while symbolizing goes freely on. In fact, every change in formulation is also a change in felt-meaning. This is necessarily so in that felt-meaning is the requisite experiential or embodied component of the meaningful. But then not every change in formulation is meaningful. A change in formulation is a change in felt-meaning only if that change is meaningful. Only if the formulation reaches and touches the felt-mass does it move it. Our formulation can be an empty abstraction or an intellectualization. It can remain disembodied in that it is not related to or relating to our felt-meaning. A disembodied formulation is in error or invalid. On the other hand, when the formulation actually touches what it is intended to symbolize the latter is changed. It is "carried forward" or advanced (p. 132, 1966). Our explication, if it actually captures felt-meaning, furthers our experiencing. The second sign of its capture, in addition to and following the felt-release, is that it changes what it seeks, through "capturing" it. Gendlin offers the following example of this, taken from a therapy setting:

If before [explicating] he struggles with "why does it make me so angry?" he now says: "I'm not really angry so much as . . . ashamed that I can't do anything in that kind of situation." . . . [And after further explication] he may say "Oh . . . it isn't so much that I'm ashamed—rather it's that I won't let myself relax because then I'll just avoid the whole thing. I keep myself at least trying to deal with it some way, by not getting over being upset about it." [p. 220 in Shlien, 1967]

This is quite an interesting state of affairs, which upon reflection, is consistent with the inherently elusive qualities of experiencing. Usually we know we have attained a phenomenon when we have staked it down, when we have photographed, catalogued, or schematized it once and for all. But in the case of experiencing or felt-meaning, when the phenomenon remains still and unmoving, when we have not "released" it and moved it, we have not yet attained it. Only when we change it, or, when it eludes us anew; only when there is a slightly different felt-bodily sense of it, have we described accurately what it was before it was carried forward.

In the setting of experiential phenomena validity or truth cannot be a question of propositional truth (p. 132, 1966). It is not a question of a match between the words with which we describe the phenomenon and the phenomenon itself. The criteria cannot be so founded because of the kind of phenomenon experiencing is. Its very nature precludes our having it at the same time we have objectified

it. We cannot both be engaged and disengaged. Further, our formulation or objectification, if it truly is that, advances our experiencing
so that it is no longer quite what it was when we first pointed at it or
lifted it out, or let it select words. Also, as we have said, experiencing
or felt-meaning is not ever a thing containing words which we
uncover or fail to uncover. Finally, although experiencing is not
indeterminate, neither is it ever fully determined. It is always only
partially formed. For these reasons and others we can never simply
superimpose the description over the phenomenon to judge their fit.

The truth of our propositions or description lies rather in other
specifiable relations between lived experience and our reflected experience of it. The character of these relations is more that of an
on-going interactive process in which either partner, the formulation
or the felt-meaning, may affect the other and in turn be affected, and
in which both partners' roles are required to create meaning. This
creative partnership, this mutually engendering two-way process never permits a static check or comparison, a matching. Our formulation
is true when it releases and carries forward that which it seeks to
express.*

An integrated experiential stance

There emerges from the features of lived experience and Gendlin's thinking a productive way to proceed. It involves a specifiable
investigatory stance which vigilantly guards against losing the phenomenon as-experienced but which allows the utilization of traditionally gathered objective data.

Earlier, drawing from several phenomenologists, we described a
general approach which does justice to the elusiveness and the
density of experiential phenomena and which contrasts clearly with
an objectivist stance. It consists in investigating phenomena unencumbered by concepts, cultural biases, or any other presumptive
views as to their nature or appearance. The goal of this stance is to
return to lived experience as it is given. It is the starting point of
most phenomenological analyses of experience and is accomplished
in Husserl's "first reduction."

From there Husserl proceeds through additional reductions to
strip experiencing and the individual experiencer of particularity. But

*The reader interested in pursuing this important question of the criteria of validity,
beyond these rudimentary points, might begin with Husserl's notion of "apodicticity" (pp.
15–16; 1970a) and Heidegger's essay "On the Essence of Truth" (pp. 292–325; 1970).

this later search for a place to stand within experiencing, what Husserl terms the "transcendental ego," is a project which does not contribute directly to the resolution of our problem. We are interested in investigations of particular phenomena, or classes of individually variable phenomena, as experienced. The most general and universal structures of experiencing are of interest to us only in that our eventual description will sit comfortably within any limits and guidelines set by that structure. In at least one way the broader and grander task of phenomenological philosophy, that of delineating general features of experience, makes a less strict procedural demand than does our problem. Given that former goal, it is sufficient to enter experiencing at any point. In the study of particular phenomena, however, we require control over access at the particular point of our interest. Further, and this is of course a problem held in common in the two types of investigations, we must have an access which permits us to make the tacit knowing of lived experience explicit.

Gendlin's description of the relation between lived and reflected experience provides precisely for this. Through direct reference we can have an initial independent access to the phenomenon of interest. By focusing on the phenomenon in its felt bodily-sense, we can then begin to explicate it. We can let words come from it, always checking back to see if the developing formulation releases the felt-meaning and advances it. The then furthered felt-meaning can be explicated afresh. The procedure generally follows this to-and-fro-movement.

With this procedure, which is a set of stances to experiencing and its formulation, we are not approaching experiencing unarmed in an effort to dwell in it no matter what it is. Clearly, given our goal, we must begin by "focusing" on the topic of our interest. We cannot search for something in particular unless we in some sense already have it. How else would we know we have found it? But just what is this starting point? Is it a topic, a word, or set of words that first interests us? And do we, armed with it, then search out the experiencing to which it might refer?

There are two possible beginnings. We might in the course of our reading light upon something that interests us. But something of interest necessarily has meaning to us. This is to say that it necessarily lifts out a particular felt-meaning. We then can have access to this felt-meaning. We can point to it as "that" and focus on it. More often than not, since what we read is generally an objectivistic literature, and therefore experientially thin, we next find ourselves saying, "no, that's not quite it." We can resume at that point the to-and-fro procedure. A second possibility is that the "topic" may be initially an experienced moment, or some aspect of several moments, that arouses our interest. It begins with, "what is that all about—and how interesting." Already we can have access to "that" and begin to explicate it.

Perhaps more typically the starting point is a combination of the two. The origin of one of the present authors' interest in introversion illustrates this. There were some recurrent aspects of his experiencing that he never put into words. At a later time these felt-meanings were lifted out while reading a section from Jung's *Psychological Types.*

There are, then, these possible origins of the problem of interest, an initial access by direct reference to it as "all of that," and a preliminary interactive process consisting of recognition, release, advance, further explication, etc. The further power of this experiential stance lies in the possibility of employing virtually any material to lift out and advance the phenomenon of interest.

Any material is fair game provided we can take an experiential stance to it with effective results. Specifically that involves letting the material function to allow us to "recognize" or lift out felt-meaning. However, even if it initially has little power to do this, if, for example, it is so abstract, or abstruse, or inconsistent that it points to nothing for us, we can still attempt an exegesis to thicken it experientially. In this way at some later point it might advance a formulation that has been developing independently of it. Our exposition in chapter 1 of Jung's theoretical writings on introversion is an instance of such an effort. In that chapter we brought together into two coherent and logically consistent models Jung's often disparate, sometimes contradictory, and generally difficult writings about introversion. In doing this, while we felt successful at that limited task, the question of experiential referents or felt-meaning for the various terms and principles of these models was one we could not answer. It was only later, well into the explication of the experience of introversion, that parts of the models began to release and add to our evolving formulation by advancing the phenomenon as-experienced. We shall demonstrate this use of the models below in the description of introversion. Our point is that, with the present procedures and experiential stances, we can approach any material that is even superficially relevant to the phenomenon of interest and treat it as a prospective formulation of it. When necessary, preparatory to this, we can put it in a form which will enhance the probability of its speaking to the phenomenon. This may involve making it as logically and systematically consistent and/or as concrete and as close to actual life situations as possible.

Another kind of material toward which we may take an experiential stance is empirically gathered data. The only additional problem posed here is that we must be able to translate it from a quantitative form to descriptive statements. Again the eventual criterion is the same as for any other material. The descriptives must advance the meaning of the particular phenomenon of interest. They are additions to our formulation if and only if they release and advance it. Empirical data has two advantages over other materials such as the theoretical or the clinical. First, of course, it is strictly governed by its own rules of procedure. It has its own controls, tests of reliability, and the like. It therefore provides us with checks over and above the kind of "experiential" validity we have described.

Second, it gives us the opportunity to design studies to answer specific questions about the phenomenon. For example, when we come across a particular aspect of it, we want to know if it is constitutive or whether it may be pared off without diminishing it. Or, we want to know if the phenomenon is manifest differently in a particular different context or if a particular feature of it is independent of context. These questions may arise directly from our experiential stance or they may be the result of reflective considerations tangential to the ongoing interactive process. As an example of the latter, we are free to raise questions suggested by any relevant literature.

In either case we can design empirical studies which will produce, or allow us to develop, relatively "thick" descriptive statements around these question areas. This material is then "testable" in terms of release and advance of the phenomenon. The TAT project, the results of which are presented in chapter 2, is an instance of an attempt to further the description of the target phenomenon in a selected domain or context. In that work we were interested primarily in clarifying the experience of introversion in interpersonal situations. This question arose in part from our observation that while previous research pointed to the salience of at least one dimension in this area (social affiliation), we were not convinced of its importance in introversion. More importantly, there was no indication in the literature of what particular form its expression might take in the experience of introversion. In part also, while we felt that there were overriding aspects peculiar to the *I*'s experience with others, we could not explicate these. By developing additional materials we hoped to be able to lift out, advance, and then make explicit these aspects. In the description of the experience of introversion below, the contribution of the construct derived from the TAT study demonstrates that we were indeed able to accomplish this.

At this point we shall relate the present method to other recent studies which attempt a rapprochement between phenomenological and empirical procedures. We hope that this will clarify further the experiential stance and its present integrative application and highlight methodological advances.

Colaizzi (in Giorgi et al., 1971), in the course of a study in which nonsense syllables were being learned, asked subjects to describe how the list "appeared" to them. By eliciting subjects' perception of the material at several criterion points in the task, Colaizzi goes beyond traditional efforts of experimentally varying types of material or conditions of learning. However, in this study as in the Van Kaam study (1966) discussed in the general introduction, while the data, or part of the data, is "experiential," the experimenter arrives at a formulation through an objectivistic stance. He gathers experiential data but he does not utilize it as such. He does not adopt an attitude or stance toward it which lets it speak to him. The experimenter, rather, attempts to keep himself out of the data and, as well, away from the phenomena. There is nothing of the dialogue which we have described between the phenomena and the data taken tentatively as its evolving formulation. The experimenter purposely restricts his insertion into the situation to that of a logical inference operator. From our point of view, this restriction diminishes the likelihood of an embodied formulation and stops short of a genuinely integrative procedure.

Another feature of the Colaizzi study is of interest. He systematically controls the situation, at least as objectively defined, to which the subjects are exposed by simply following a standardized design. There is a danger here in the way in which we utilize this well-developed feature of empirical method. We must be careful not to take the situation as a definition of the phenomenon of interest. More precisely, the phenomenon of interest cannot be defined as the

response to the experimenter's arrangement, no matter how in-
formed that arrangement might be. Since experiencing—the target
phenomenon here—is in part a meaning-giving, we cannot exclusively
anchor it to a particular situation to which only it ultimately can give
a meaning. The locus of definition cannot be that of a stimulus
chaining its response. The anchor is the subject's perception of the
situation, since only that is the phenomenon itself. The experience of
learning, for example, is not whatever occurs in a situation objectively defined as a learning situation. Nor is it even whatever occurs
in the presence of behavior defined by the experimenter as an
instance of learning. Clearly, the subject may "learn" a given number
of nonsense syllables and have no experience of learning anything.

The empirical method, then, offers in standardized and controlled situations a feature which an integrated procedure may assimilate but only with modification. The experimentally manipulated
situation may function as an immediate or likely occasion of the
phenomenon, but not as its definitive or necessary precursor. It may
be, only, more or less evocative.

Colaizzi's effort limits the role of the experimenter and limits, as
well, the role of experience itself to an additional variable intended
to clarify the focal empirical findings within an essentially objectivistic paradigm. Fischer (in Giorgi et al., 1971) advances beyond
Colaizzi when she clearly takes an experiential stance to the phenomenon of interest, here the experience of privacy. A number of other
researchers (Buckley in Giorgi et al., 1971; Romanyshyn in Giorgi)
proceed exclusively in this way which they refer to as a dialogic or
dialectic or reflective method. As we have indicated, Gendlin's work
and our adaptation of it to research in personality provide a needed
description of this stance. The dialogue is understandable in terms of
the complex interaction between felt-meaning and its explicit formulation.

Fischer, in these terms, begins by attempting to capture her own
sense of being in private. She allows the explicit topic to lift out an
only tacit sense of the phenomenon, initially in concrete instances
from her own life. She lets words come from the concrete instance,
utilizing the experiential check given to her with the evolving formulation.

In the Fischer study, however, there is an important integrative
feature complementing the experimenter's experiential posture. She
asks a group of student subjects, and eventually a second group, to

recall and describe instances of being in private. They then, together with the experimenter, arrive at a description which has consensual validity in addition to apodictic certainty. This is an advance over those studies in which the experimenter rests entirely on his own intuition and reflection. It is an integration that borrows design procedures from empiricism which the latter takes as critical, repeatability and generality. It incorporates them without relinquishing its own criteria.

Stevick (in Giorgi et al., 1971) brings together some of the features of the Fischer study with some of those of Colaizzi. She begins with semistructured interviews with subjects. The interviews are standardized in a way which allows subjects to amplify their experience within directions set by themselves. The investigator then abstracts themes from the protocols and fits all the components into a single extensive description. Only at this point does she assume an experiential stance over against this description, taking it as "all of that" that is the phenomenon of interest. In this way she combines empirical and phenomenological procedures to arrive at an embodied formulation.

These studies are representative of current efforts to evolve an experiential method, one which remains true to the phenomenon as experienced. They clearly seek to rest the investigation on both subjects' and experimenters' experience as ultimate sources of the phenomenon. Central to this method is an experiential stance, a dialogic posture to the phenomenon by the investigator, by subjects, or by both. In fact, more generally, there is a tendency in this method for the roles of the subject and the experimenter to blur, since it is recognized that they are both equally legitimate sources of the phenomenon. On the one hand the subject is not deceived, he does not remain immersed as an unreflecting object for the experimenter. On the other hand, the investigator does not attempt to remain completely unimbedded as if he were outside the laboratory at the controls, neutral, uninterested, or uninvolved in his own project.

At the same time, however, there is a trend to integrate this budding phenomenological method with empirical procedures or modifications of them. It is being recognized that at various stages the empirical method actually can facilitate attainment of the descriptive formulation and can add its own power to that formulation. For example, the controlled situation of the experimental method can be utilized for its evocative power, recognizing, again, that the manipulated situation functions only to conjure up and delimit the phenomenon, not to define it.

Second, there is beginning to emerge in these studies the suggestion that the empirical method, particularly its rules of statistical validity, can be utilized in those stages of an investigation prior to the assumption of an experiential stance. For example, material generated in the analysis of protocols of subjects may be governed by traditional rules of evidence.

Within this context we can review our method in the present project. In chapter 1 we have analyzed Jung's theoretical and descriptive writings on introversion and presented them in a form which allows fruitful reflection on them. Our posture in that analysis was not yet the experiential one we have described above. At that point, we were not attempting to create a dialogue with whatever tacit sense of the phenomenon we might have had. Our exegesis, rather, sought first to clarify the theoretical structure in its own terms. In the course of this exegesis, we revealed the Cartesian bias in the theory, the heavy use of analogy to physical systems, in short, the reductionistic tendency; while "rediscovering" and gaining added respect for the equally weighty experiential bedrock of Jung's thought. We arrived at two models which economically synthesized and accounted for the theoretical material. Second, we asked the limited question both of the theoretical and of the more descriptive material: To what in experience do they point? With these two procedures, again, we were developing material for an eventual dialogue. As we have indicated, it is part of the power of a phenomenological method that it can be applied to a broader range of material. In fact, herein lies a key to its potential for integration with other methods.

In chapter 2 we moved from theoretical material based on clinical insight to an empirical data-gathering format. Through this second project we developed additional material toward which we could take an experiential stance. A controlled stimulus situation was selected which would further the description of introversion in the interpersonal domain. The situation was chosen also for its semistructured properties. This gave to subjects an opportunity to express their views of interpersonal relations and of their world more generally in a relatively open and yet standardized situation. Protocols were sorted through the intuitive judgment of one of the authors.

While the sort clearly was based on an as yet inexplicit sense of the target phenomenon, the judgments at that stage were set completely within an empirical procedure. We relied on traditional empirical criteria of evidence, not yet on an apodictic check. We have described the details of that procedure in the methods section of chapter 2. It involves abstracting rules from the sorted protocols. The posture of the abstracter remains objective in the sense that he looks for any commonality which accurately sorts the protocols within an accepted level of statistical significance. He attempts to stay, for the moment, outside of his own sense of the target phenomenon and open, therefore, to any features of the protocols. This is, of course, a tried and true empirical approach. Through it we arrived at a set of empirically reliable rules based on an as yet to be explicated sense of the phenomenon.

Our review of the literature in phenomenological psychology should make it clear that there is in the present study an advance toward a genuine and powerful integration not only of empirical method but of clinical evidence as well with phenomenological method. We have two models of the phenomenon, each the result of a logically and internally consistent exegesis of theory which is itself grounded in clinical experience. Further, we have a set of rules which are empirically reliable and which are open to experimental validation. At the same time these rules are themselves based on an intuitive judgment which is no less than the tacit sense of the phenomenon in a person intimately familiar with it.

It is these two sets of material to which we apply the phenomenological method. They both serve as tentative formulations which are taken over against all of that that is the felt-meaning of introversion. In this way both the clinical-theoretical insights and the empirically gathered data become an integral part of an interactive partnership between the advancing felt-meaning and its evolving formulation. This we offer as a truly integrative methodology.

Another gain in the present work is that we have explicitly described an experiential stance. Terms such as "dialogue" and "reflection" are given an experiential thickness and clear experiential referents through the description earlier of the dialectic relation between felt-meaning and evolving formulation, or more generally, between lived and reflected experience. To reiterate, the present method is a modification of most philosophical phenomenological procedures in that the vehicle of a presuppositionless entry into experiencing which leads to its general structure is replaced by the possibility of continually fresh access to a specified phenomenon-as-experienced. Such access is critical and forms the methodological basis of a phenomenological psychology. Again, the experiential stance provides intrinsically an apodictic check which we have also described in experiential terms. Given the integrative potential of the present method, then, validity may depend on both phenomenological and empirical criteria. Or, as in the present investigation, the eventual formulation can have the persuasive power lent by the confluence of (1) a collection of clinical insights fashioned into theoretical models, (2) a set of empirical data translated, by inference, into a construct, and (3) the experiential stance wherein both of these serve as tentative formulations.

Another feature of the present investigation, added here incidentally, although it might well be recognized more formally as an important feature of the method, is the fact of two investigators. The experiential stance here is a dialogue in a double sense. Added to the interaction between felt-meaning and formulation is the possibility that any of the several functional relationships in that partnership (recognition, lifting out, advancing, etc.) may be provided at any point by either member of the investigatory team.

Of course, while we are excited about the efficacy and power of this integrated method, a final test is the capacity of the formulation to lift and advance the particular phenomenon for the reader. Ultimately, the validity of the present descriptive formulation of introversion rests with the reader. This is not offered as a rhetorical flourish but is, in a sense, a real difference between a phenomenological and an empirical method. In an exclusively empirical investigation, the validity of an obtained relation between variables holds even if it says nothing to the reader, fails to advance his understanding, remains outside or even contrary to his experience. It can be valid even in the instance where it remains disembodied, that is, meaningless to him. Where, however, as in the present method, the object of the study is a formulation of a phenomenon-as-experienced, that formulation must speak to the phenomenon for the reader. While there is a check inherent in the process of formulation, the generality of the description waits finally for the reader. It must embody and advance his experience. It must touch him. If it is not meaningful to him, there is no remnant sense in which it is true.

In the present study, then, the loci of validity are complex. The construct of introversion consisting of seven rules is an empirical finding. The rules are reliable in the empirical sense of that term, i.e., they are, presumably, repeatable. The formulation based on these rules, on the two models of introversion derived from Jung, and on these two taken as tentative formulations over against the only felt-meaning of the phenomenon is important in another sense. It provides for us a reasonably complete expression of the experience of introversion. Its final validity is a function of its evocative power for the reader.

The description of the core of this phenomenological method, the discussion of its possible integration with other approaches, and, of course, the present example of its application, may serve to dispel the mystification which generally surrounds the experiential method. We hope to have demonstrated (1) that phenomenology is not soft, fuzzy, and intuitive, in the sense of unclear as to what it entails; but that, on the contrary, it is engrossed in a fruitful clarification of how its own approach and, as importantly, how other approaches are constituted; (2) that it is not itself guilty, ironically, of its own charge to others of being disembodied, abstract, and jargon-laden; (3) that it has application to personality and psychology generally; and, finally, (4) that its understanding of objectivism as only one possible view of reality is a critique which does not preclude a constructive alliance.

Jung, I/E, and the "middle term"

There is one more item of unfinished business which will serve conveniently as a transition from methodological issues to their application to the experience of introversion. It may have become evident to the reader at a number of points that our presentation of a phenomenological method and descriptions of the structure of experience seem to involve the same issue with which Jung grapples in his investigation of I/E, namely, the role of the subject and object in perception or consciousness. This parallel is not accidental. It raises the following question or questions: What is the relation between Jung's insight into the I/E difference and his method of dealing with it, and the structure of experience and the present experiential method of studying I/E differences?

The section on Gendlin's work demonstrated the difficulties in eventually describing experience due to its tacit and elusive nature.

The section prior to it suggested, through a description of lived experience, its often ambiguous and seemingly contradictory character. We noted in passing some of these antinomies inherent in experiencing. To reiterate, it is both constituted, already there, as when we already have the rear of the house when perceiving it from the front; and it is constituting, it is a building up of our world. Lived experience is both immediately given to us, since we are embedded in the world; and it is a construction, it is created by us. Experience is world-disclosing and, at the same time, we are the world we disclose. Or in existential terms experiencing has both a "thrownness" and a "project." We are beings placed in, threaded to the world and yet we are always our projects, what we are intending or choosing to be.

Erwin Straus points to an additional enigma or ambiguity belonging particularly to sensory experiencing. We shall quote it here since it plays a role in our description of introversion to follow:

The observed happenings are at once part of him, who has seen them, and no part of him, for they are the Other, the object of his observations. [May, 1967, p. 148]

These antinomies, referred to by Straus as the "logically offensive" character of lived experience, as well as the complexity of the relationship between lived experience and our reflections on it, have made description difficult.

The traditional "resolution" to these problems for logical or post-conceptual thinking has been to assume the Cartesian dualisms. The inability to grasp how experience and the person is both in-the-world and world-creating has led to the assumption of the disembodied subject, the worldless subject and/or of the subjectless world, the passive sensorial respondent. We have mentioned Van Kaam's point that there are generally two classes of theory in psychology. One class is more or less exclusively intrapsychic, subjectivistic, the other extrapsychic, mechanistic, and objectivistic. Both deny the enigmatic and logically offensive quality of experiencing. They are born of the two sides of these antinomies, yet they fail to conceptualize or describe experience in a way which, true to experience, captures the ambiguities. They do not approach a consideration of the experiencing person in the world.

In this general context we must consider Jung. As a student of philosophy he observed the bifurcation in prephenomenological phi-

losophies, the idealisms and the realisms. He also saw parallel dichotomies in literature and in psychology (Freud and Adler). Jung
connected the fact of these warring factions in various systems of
thought to an observation in his clinical practice of the existence of
two general personality types among his patients. His hypothesis was
that conceptual systems are split in twos because there are two
classes of individuals, introverts and extraverts. In this manner he
"psychologized" Western thought.

Unfortunately, however, his methodology trips on the same
dualistic thinking which was the basis for his insight into personality.
Both his theories and his descriptions of the phenomena assume the
split between subject and object, between psyche or consciousness
and body or world. Van Kaam considers Jung's theories subjectivistic
in that they are intrapsychic (p. 209, 1966). We are in agreement
with this. Consciousness is inside the head for Jung. But beyond this
internal location, his theories are objectivistic. The phenomena of
interest, although he refers to them as attitudes or views, are treated
as things. They are given the properties of things and are approached
and described as if they were things. They are domains intimately
related to other domains, they are systems with certain energic
properties. It is to Jung's credit that he did recognize I/E as attitudinal postures, as differing pervasive views toward the world. He did
not reduce them to the simplistic and desiccated inside/outside
distinctions of later researchers. But because the underpinnings of his
methods were essentially objectivistic, he never approached the attitudes as such in his writings. The phenomenon of introvertedness, a
particular embodied posture, a particular mode of being-in-the-world,
remains largely untouched by Jung. Jung could not accomplish a
description of introvertedness because he had at his service only
reductionistic methods. He had approaches that dealt only with the
logically offensive character of experiencing and with its elusiveness
in the face of reflected thought by assuming a split between subject
and object, between observer and the observed.

Phenomenology discovers these ambiguities and captures by description the logically offensive features of experience. It is a method
which cuts through the Cartesian derived presumption of observer/
observed separability. The subject/object split is transcended as experience is allowed to emerge as what it is—a being absorbed in the
"other." Both in the phenomenological method and in its product, a

description of experience, there is a bridging of this and other postconceptual dichotomies. Experience and the person as "being-in-the-world" are the "middle term" (Merleau-Ponty, 1962, p. 77).

Our method of approaching problems in personality is phenomenological. We take it to be true of every person that he is an experiencing being, a being-in-the-world. His personality is a particular mode of being-in-the world.

With respect to the present problem of I/E, our thesis is that some apparently contradictory features of experiencing, some "oppositions," provide a ground for this particular difference among people. A person consistently accentuates, or rather a person is in his being an accentuation of one or the other side of these "contradictions." For example, a person consistently emphasizes in his experiencing the "part of him" aspect of observed happenings as opposed to the "no part of him"; or a person emphasizes the meaning-giving aspect while another accentuates the "already there" aspect of experiencing, the meaning as immanent in the moment. We shall find, then, in the introverted mode of being a tacit but consistent "resolution" of these antinomies.

A possible point of confusion is that the tacit resolutions which constitute introversion and extraversion respectively remain, nonetheless, modes of being-in-the-world. While the contradictory features are the very ones which occasioned the twin reductions of objectivistic and subjectivistic theories, they also are the ground of the two modes, I/E. In fact, the two modes of being are, respectively, the tacit or lived sense of the twin reduction. As particular modes of being, they remain like any others styles of experiencing which, as such, require a phenomenological method to be explicated. Whatever is the peculiarly introverted aspect of the I's experiencing, it still has the structure of experience—it is still both immediately given and yet necessarily a construal by him, etc.

A final point confirms, rightly so, our debt to Jung rather than our critique of him. For it is as students of personality, but more particularly of Jung's theory of personality, that we are enabled to add to a general phenomenology the idea of typology. We posit, guided by Jung, a region of phenomena intermediate in range of variability between the invariant structure of experience and the continuous flux of individual experience from moment to moment. This is the traditional region of typological theory. We find, then, within lived experience additional aspects that are relatively stable for a class of individuals. These constitute the experience of introversion.

In summary: (1) There is in the structure of experience a set of seemingly contradictory aspects which give rise to two variant models of being-in-the-world termed "introversion" and "extraversion"; and (2) Jung's insight into I/E is based on the observation of postconceptual manifestations of these structures.

4. The Experience of Introversion

Introduction

Phenomenology emphasizes how much is experiential in our words, yet lost as such in our words. If we write, "It was an engaging book," we generally read this phrase as less than it was in experience. We reduce it to the thought that the book was satisfactory. This is not simply because we are only reading the words and not having the experience that called them forth. It is also because we can easily lose the experiential basis of words. What do we have to write or rather what do we have to read to recapture what it was to find a book "engaging"? If we write, "It *attracted* me and *held* me in its influence and power; it *bound* me to it; it *engrossed* me; it *occupied* me; I *participated* in it,"* (emphasis added) we perhaps begin to recapture what was meant by the original phrase. We ask the reader of the following description of introversion to attempt to let its words speak to him in their fullest or experientially thickest sense. This involves taking a posture which allows the words to move him, to be concretely felt by him; it involves participating in them and being occupied by them.

There is another difficulty to be avoided in verbal description. Unlike a canvas where what is seen is seen all at once, verbal description operates in linear time. Its message necessarily unfolds gradually. Pieces must be held in mind and fitted together through the course of the description. Further, while the proximity of the forms on a canvas implies connectedness, in an essay it is difficult not to have temporal proximity imply cause and effect. We ask the reader to approach the following description as a picture.

Our description is organized primarily under four headings; the *I*'s lived experience, the *I*'s reflected experience, the *I*'s views of self, and the experience of the *I* with another person. In the course of the description, four major connections are drawn between the experience of introversion and the two models of chapter 1 and the two central findings of chapter 2. They are: (1) Some features of the *I*'s lived experience provide the experiential referents of Jung's struc-

Webster's Seventh New Collegiate Dictionary (1963), s.v. "engage."

tural model of introversion; (2) Some features of the *I*'s reflected experience provide the experiential referents of Jung's energy model of introversion; (3) The features of the *I*'s experience which constitute "self-concern" are described; (4) The *I*'s interpersonal sense of "distance" is further clarified by examining it in the general context of the *I*'s experience with another person.

Lived Experience

Sense of lived experience as mediated

We begin by describing some characteristics of the *I*'s lived experience from an example. There is a small party of people some of whom are *I*s and some *E*s. They are on an outing and are hiking. They have been climbing and have just come to a clearing where they look out upon a panoramic view. It is exhilarating and engaging. It is a lived moment for each member of the party.

Our problem is to distinguish the lived experience of the *I*s from that of the *E*s. What invariant aspects of this moment are peculiarly introverted? There are two truisms one might apply to the mountain scene to help us identify an overriding introverted characteristic.

The first is that all of the sights in the mountain panorama are the same, the green and wooded valley below, the birds gliding in the thermals, the mist over the distant mountains. This moment contains these particular objects which can be perceived by any observer. But a second truism is equally applicable. Each individual in the party experiences the scene somewhat differently. Each individual brings to it different interests and needs, a different history, even a different perceptual apparatus; each views the scene from a different vantage point. The bird-watcher sees a "new" bird for his life-list; the depressed individual senses his insignificance and loneliness in the enormity of the valley; and the lover sees that the world is love.

Let us consider the possibility that two classes of individuals on the mountain, *I*s and *E*s, differ in their utilization of one or the other of these truisms. The *I* is directed toward the differentness of his experience; while the *E* emphasizes the sameness of the sight. How are these different emphases experienced?

The *I*, who focuses on differentness, is feeling that his experience at that moment in the clearing is changed in his experiencing it. It is changed in that it is he who is experiencing it. Part of what is given to him in the moment is a sense that by experiencing it, that which he is experiencing is being changed. Part of what is exhilarating or elating to the *I* as he confronts the mountain panorama is his sense that his experience is changing through the fact of his experiencing it. His emphasis on the individualized nature of experience is sensed in experience in this way. There is for the *I* what we will refer to as a sensed mediated aspect of his lived experience. It is as though what he receives in the moment is a version or a rendering or an instant recounting of the moment. It is sensed as a recounting or a retelling in that it is other than the event or the moment itself. It is sensed as changed. It is as if a difference exists between what is "there" and what is experienced, and the *I* perceives this difference in his experiencing. The precise experience of the difference is his sense that what he experiences is changing through his experiencing of it. We are not saying that the object of his perception, the scene itself, is sensed as changing but rather that the *I*'s experience of the lived moment has this mediated aspect, a sense of his experience, given in the moment, "as-changed."

How is it for the *E*? The *E*, the focuser on sameness, is feeling that what he is experiencing in the lived moment is more directly the sights themselves. His experience is sensed as a direct copy or reflection of the mountain scene. His emphasis on the sameness of the sight and his lack of emphasis on the individualized nature of his experience has this directly given quality. Let us call it a sense of a presentative aspect of the lived moment. There is nothing of the peculiarly introverted sense of what he experiences as changed by his experiencing of it. The *E*'s exhilaration in the mountain scene is simply the finding and the "having," in the experiential sense, of something in the world that is what it is, exhilarating, beautiful, or the like.

These two alternative aspects of lived experience we are describing imply no consistent differences in content between the lived experience of the *I* and that of the *E*. The content of the *I*'s lived moment, if we could measure it from some objective point of view, is not more changed, original, creative, whimsical, or even richer than is the *E*'s. It is not more individualized or personalized in any substantive way. Conversely, the content of the *E*'s lived experience is not more directly reflective of the moment. If we could measure it, we would not find it a more accurate or valid picture of what is "real" in the mountain scene. Rather, the I's lived experience is distinguished from the E's by an overriding aspect of it: the sense of it as being changed through his experience of it, or, for the E, the sense of it as directly given. For one there is the sense of it as "other than"; for the other there is the sense of it as "the same as." The difference we are describing is a difference in a compelling aspect or quality of lived experience. We are not arguing here that this difference is reflected in any other more objective or more substantive or more behavioral aspect of the I's personality or activity.

We are describing a differential aspect of lived experience. The I's sense of his experience as mediated and the E's sense of his as presentative are themselves part of their lived experience. Neither aspect of felt-experience is directly dependent on later reflection. Neither requires a pointing at self in relation to the object or scene, or a making of the felt-aspect explicit. Both aspects are felt in the moment as part of the moment.

But while it is primarily an experiential difference that we are describing, recognition of the I's sensed mediated nature of his experience is crucial to a more general understanding of the introverted way of being in the world. It is also a major building block in our description of introversion.

The description thus far centers on the role of the subject and object in perception, a problem which was Jung's starting point in the development of the distinction between I and E. The truisms which were employed to introduce the present aspect of experience may also be seen as respective slogans for the two bases of phenomenal reality, the subject and the object. The first is a statement of the personal nature of the world of our consciousness. It is a slogan for a perspectival view of reality (Merleau-Ponty, 1963, p. 186). The second is a statement of the constancy of the objects of our consciousness, the fixity and concrete identity of the world for all observers. It is a slogan for a naturalistic or objectivist view of reality. Reality is what is out there. It is constituted by the objects in the world.

We will say more below about how these aspects of experience provide a fitting experiential referent for Jung's "solution" to the role of the subject and object in consciousness as articulated in his structural model. But first, we shall turn to the description of two additional aspects of lived experience.

Sense of lived experience as mine

If the *I*, who focuses on the individualized nature of experience, feels that his experience of the moment is changing through his experience of it, then he must feel it is his, uniquely a part of him. It owes its particular existence to him. It is his possession and his product and is experienced as *mine*.

We are beginning to describe one side of a variable aspect of experience, namely the felt-source of one's experience. The two possible sources are the self and the world, or the self and the "other." These are logically an inclusive set, and, both logically and experientially, mutually exclusive with reference to a particular given moment.

A further understanding of the felt-source of experience may be gained by turning to the *E*. If the *E* feels his experience is a direct reflection of the scene and not mediated by his experiencing of it, then the felt-source of his experience is more the scene or object of perception itself. The felt-source is the other's or the object's. From the point of view of his experience of the moment, the *E* is feeling that it is "the other's"; it is not me, not part of me. It is "the object's."

The second characteristic of the *I*'s lived moment is this sense of the felt-mineness of his experience in the moment. What we are pointing to in experience with this variable of mineness is both difficult to grasp and central in reaching an understanding of the experience of the *I*. Let us again turn to examples to bolster the description.

This first example will need subsequently to be qualified but the example together with its qualifications will help us on our way. The setting is a lecture hall, a group discussion, or any context in which you are being exposed to the ideas of other people. The topic is of interest to you and you become engaged as the speaker presents his argument. Some of his points are new to you and exciting. But there is an elation associated with your experience that is other than the excitement of the novel or the surge from intellectual stimulation. It is the feeling that the thought or idea that you are taking away from the lecture is yours. From your point of view, if you are an *I*, it is felt as "mine." We do not mean simply that it is mine in the sense that it is something that you did not have a moment ago and now you have. It is sensed as mine in that it is not the other person's.

Even though you just heard it from the mouth of another, it feels as if it were yours.

Again, the *I*'s emphasis on the mediated nature of his lived experience makes it feel like it is his. He has changed it in his experiencing of it and the changing of it makes it his. His experience of this felt-source is a sense of the mineness of his experience.

This example of the *I*'s experience during an engaging lecture requires two qualifications before it can stand as illustrative of this aspect of the *I*'s lived experience more generally. The first qualification has to do with the following question: Exactly what is it that is felt as mine by the *I* in the moment (or by the *E* as the other's)? The example suggests that it is a discrete element such as an idea or a feeling or a sensation that is experienced as mine. More generally, however, what is sensed as mine by the *I* in the moment is the experience-as-a-whole. Part of the *I*'s experience of the moment is the sense that the experience in its entirety is his.

The second qualification is clarified by the first. In the example of the lecture, the source of that which is experienced as mine is patent. It is another person. There is unambiguously in the situation an author of the thought or idea. More generally, however, and particularly if it is not a discrete element but the experience-as-a-whole which is experienced as mine, this sense of the source of the experience occurs in contexts in which the source is not so clear or unambiguous. It occurs more typically in situations where a dimension of mine/other's is apparently of little salience. It is a more subtle aspect of the experience in this latter context. Unlike our lecture example, the sense of mineness does not usually occur in contexts in which it might appropriately be accompanied by a sense of plagiarism.

Having clarified the context in which this sense of mineness occurs, let us return to our friends looking out at the mountain panorama. Here the source of that which is experienced is ambiguous and of little salience. There is no lecturer presenting results of work from his own laboratory. The mountain panorama is everybody's and nobody's. Now the *I*, as we have said, accentuates the individualized nature of experience rather than the constancy or identity of the objects of experience. One way in which this focus is realized in experience is that the moment in its entirety is felt as mine. For the *E*, his focus on the sameness or identity is realized in experience as the sense that all that is the experience of the moment has its source in the object, in the mountain panorama.

The sense of mineness for the *I* is constitutive of his lived experience. The depressed individual, the bird watcher, the lover, each enthralled in his own way with the view from the mountain, senses the experience as mine if he is an *I*. In lived experience what is experienced is given in the moment. It is given in the relation between the individual and the world. For the *I* there is this additional but also given sense of the mineness of the experience. The sense of mineness does not emerge from and is not dependent on a later reflection on the moment. Not only does the *I* not sense that a particular entity within the experience is mine, he does not as part of the experience of mineness raise the question of mineness. It is, again, part of the given experience-as-a-whole.

This last is no doubt confusing. The sense of mineness is a given part of a particular engaged experience; but it is, at the same time, a sensed characteristic of that moment. It is a part of it and yet a kind of immediately given view of it, a sense as to its source. The experience-as-a-whole for the *I* is sensed as mine, and part of the given experience-as-a-whole is its mineness.

We will give one final example or parallel to help clarify this sense of the felt-source of one's lived experience. It is more precisely a parallel than an example since we are going to ask the *I* and *E* to put into words their felt-experiences of a particular lived moment. Let us compare the experience of an *I* and an *E* on the Rorschach Inkblot Test. Let us assume that both are relatively unsophisticated psychologically. They have completed the task, having given a number of responses or percepts. Now we want them to reflect on what they were experiencing when they were engaged with the inkblots. We ask them how they view the percepts that each has given. In particular, we ask what they see as the source of the percepts. The *I* might say something closer to: I thought about the castle after I saw what could be taken as a huge door knob. Something in the card would stimulate my imagination. The *E*, however, might say: Well, I saw those things on the cards because they are there. Sometimes they were more difficult to find but if you kept looking you would see them.

With this parallel, we have completed the presentation of this second aspect of the *I*'s lived experience. Again, it should be clear that this variable aspect of lived experience brings us back to Jung's starting point: the fact of the subject and object as the two necessary bases of consciousness. The felt-source of one's experience is an experiential counterpart of the differential weighting of the roles of the subject and object in consciousness. The individual who senses the experience as mine is weighting or emphasizing the role of the subject or, in Jung's terms, the "subjective determinants" of consciousness; while the individual who is experiencing the source as the object's is emphasizing the "objective determinants."

We have, then, that part of the experience of being subjectively oriented, of being an *I*, is the sense of the mineness of one's experience and of one's experience as changing or being mediated through the experiencing of it.

Sense of lived experience as exclusive possession

A third characteristic of lived experience follows quite directly from the first two. For the *I*, if what he is experiencing is changing through his experiencing of it and if it is felt to be his in origin, then it is felt as unshared. Only he is changing it in this way. Only he is having this particular experience. The *I* is feeling that it is mine and that it is not the other's. It is mine only. A part of the *I*'s lived moment is this sense of the exclusive mineness of his experience.

The *I* feels that what he is experiencing is not being and cannot be experienced by another in the same way. Not only is the experience felt to be unshared by another, the *I* also feels that he is not sharing and cannot share the other's experience. He senses in his given experience that no one is empathizing with it at the moment and that it is not itself a product of his empathizing with someone else.

Conversely what the *E* experiences is sensed as more directly what is in the scene. He feels that what others are experiencing is the same thing. A prominent characteristic of his lived experience is a sense that what he is experiencing is being shared. If we were to make explicit the *E*'s felt experience in our mountain panorama example, he might be thinking that all on the mountain are having the same experience. The mountain panorama is the mountain panorama. What is being experienced in this moment is what one experiences in such moments, and others here are experiencing it also. His emphasis on sameness is experienced as a sense of the sharedness of his experience. The *I*, on the other hand, is having an experience that is more consistent with the thought that what is being experienced is fashioned by the fact of my experiencing it. Hence, what I am experiencing no one else is experiencing. It is my experience and mine only.

The sense of mineness and exclusive possession are important as central parts of the *I*'s lived experience. However, while the sense of mineness is accompanied by the present unshared and private quality, this is not to say that it is sensed as internally located or as "in-me." The conceptual framework "in/out," which has been so popular in various I/E measures and I/E related variables, is not descriptive of the experience of introversion. Experience, generally, has an "in-the-world" quality. This is to say that it is not sensed as "in-me." Second, the present sense of exclusive possession does not imply that introversion involves a sense of one's experience as being given by or as associated with an inner world or unconscious domain. It is not sensed as emanating from some hypothetical psychic structure. It is easy to mistake here the conceptual or theoretical for the experiential. Jung, as we saw in chapter 1, associated introversion in one of his models with a particular psychic domain. But he did not state, in fact he explicitly denied, that it is part of the *I*'s experience to be aware of this association. The point we are trying to underline is that introvertedness is linked in the popular mind with the "inner world" and this erroneously implies that the *I* senses his experience or his world as internal, or "inner," or cut off from the rest of the world. He does not, as we shall have occasion to point out again in other contexts. The sense of privateness or unsharedness of the *I*'s lived moment is experienced as a feeling of exclusive possession, not of internal location or of out-of-this-world location.

But earlier we have described "being-in-the-world" as a general quality of all lived experience. Is this not antithetical to our description of the introvert's sense of lived experience as one's exclusive possession? Can it be both in-the-world and felt as unshared or private?

To answer this question we need to review a bit. The lived moment involves being engaged with the world in such a way that any sensed split between subject and object is transcended. Being engaged is an encounter which is the given psychological reality. It is what is experienced. For the *I*, however, what is given in the encounter is additionally sensed as being given exclusively to him. "Encounter," as used here, is a general term for a meeting in which there is a transcendence or forgetting of self by either of the principals involved. As we use the term, any lived moment necessarily involves an encounter. For the *I*, too, there is this forgetting of self, but the particular experience is sensed as being his experience only. The given experience-as-a-whole in being engaged with the other is sensed as changed in his experiencing of it, and changed toward his peculiar version of the moment. It is sensed as an unshared version. This is easy to understand in the instance of an encounter between a person and a book, or between a person and the remote lecturer of an earlier example. Although these others together with the person constitute the world of that moment, they cannot be felt by the person to share his given experience of their encounter. But in the instance of an encounter composed of two people in a heated discussion, it is not so clear. Here we will need to distinguish between kinds of encounter, between the genuine or authentic and the inauthentic, where the former approaches a mutually shared experience of the moment.

Let us defer the discussion of an encounter between two people for a later section of this chapter. At that point we will clarify what it is like for an *I* to encounter another person. Here we can only reassert that while the lived moment is in-the-world, the feeling of the *I* in such a moment is that it is mine, my exclusive and unshared possession. Engagement in the world and the sense of exclusiveness are not antithetical. Further, this sense of unsharedness is descriptive only of immediate experience. Upon reflection or in reflected experience the *I* does feel as if he can and in fact is prone to share his "experience" with others, as we will subsequently describe.

Experiential referents: Lived experience and the structural model

We have described three characteristics of the *I*'s lived experience as distinguished from that of the *E*'s. Additionally, we have indicated how these aspects of experience are consonant with Jung's idea that the role of the subject and object in consciousness is basic to the distinction between introversion and extraversion. Now we shall discuss more specifically how the peculiarly introverted qualities of the *I*'s lived experience provide experiential referents for one of Jung's two models of introversion, the structural model. Also, we shall begin to develop ties between the experiential description given thus far and the empirical findings presented in chapter 2.

Let us recall that in the structural model Jung dealt with the problem of the subjective and objective determinants of consciousness by positing two psychic domains in each individual, one housing objective determinants, the other subjective determinants. Introversion is defined as an attitude resulting from reliance on a subjective view, extraversion a reliance on an objective view. A central idea governing the model is that of correspondence. The attitude resulting from input from the subjective domain is said by Jung to correspond less accurately with the objective stimulus occasioning the view. How is this experienced by the introvert?

It is our belief that the answer to such questions lies in the examination of the salient aspects of experiencing. We are less prone to believe that degree of correspondence will be clearly reflected in objective measures of the content of experience.

We assert that the experiential referent of Jung's concept of lack of correspondence is the I's sense that what he is experiencing in the moment is changed through his experiencing of it. If it has been changed, it does not correspond. This "changed" aspect is a cornerstone of the experience of introversion and implies further a sense of the moment as mine, exclusively and unshared.

For the E, on the other hand, correspondence is reflected by experiencing the lived moment as directly given by the object, more like a copy of the object or the object itself, or a mirror held up to the moment. With the object as its source it feels like an experience that is also given to others, that is shared.

We have in the above arrived at the felt-source, the sense of mine/other's, indirectly by way of the relation of the idea of correspondence to the mediated/presentative aspect of experience. Returning to Jung's model once again, we can derive the differences in felt-source more directly. In addition to correspondence, the structural model distinguishes the introverted and extraverted views by positing different loci of origin for them. This already points to a difference in felt-source as an experiential referent. The introverted view is thought to originate in a domain which is more or less autonomous of and removed from the immediate objective situation, the "external world." It comes from a hypothesized unconscious domain of which Jung states the I is not aware. If source is salient, and the source is neither the world nor some internal domain, some sense of location "in-me," then the source is felt simply as mine.

Incidentally, that a central aspect of the I's lived moment involves this distinction in the experience of possession (mine or the other's) is also implied in Straus's statement discussed earlier in the section on "phenomenology." His description of the ambiguity inherent in the nature of experience, which Jung intuited was the basis of the I/E distinction, is roughly as follows: Experience is "at once part of him" who is experiencing it, and "no part of him," for it is "the Other." The I/E distinction relates to this ambiguity as follows: The *I* is oriented to the "part of him" side of the ambiguity and experiences this as a sense of mineness. The *E* resolves the ambiguity by orienting toward the "no part of him" pole which is accompanied by the sense of the experience as belonging to the other or the object.

In addition to these connections with Jung's theory of introversion and the structure of experience derived from phenomenological psychology, lines may also be drawn between the salient characteristics of the *I*'s lived experience and empirical results obtained through the analysis of fantasy productions of *I*s and *E*s. Starting with the theme of interpersonal distance, if part of what the *I* is experiencing is sensed as changing as he experiences it, and thus unshared, unique to him, there is implicit in this nexus a sense of interpersonal distance from the other. Within this framework the prominence of a theme of distance between individuals becomes understandable.

It should be clear that we are not saying that a sense of distance is part of the *I*'s lived experience. It is not. Distance between self and other is not felt in an engaged moment. We are simply indicating how the present aspects of the *I*'s lived experience logically approach a theme of distance found in the TAT stories of *I*s. In the discussion of reflected experience we shall describe how this theme of distance, expressed in fantasy, is experienced by the *I*.

In a similar vein the reason for the salience of the theme of self-concern, the second theme found in the TATs of *I*s, is illuminated by the present description of the *I*'s lived experience. The *I*'s sense of the mineness of his experience ineluctably produces a salience of self or concerns with self. The experience of this self-concern, like distance, is more properly a part of the *I*'s reflected experience and will be developed in the next section.

To close this section, we will attempt to establish the web which connects the two TAT themes. The focus of the introvert on the individualized or personalized nature of experience is given in the lived moment as the sense of his experience as mediated. This sense of his experience as changing through his experiencing of it is inextricably related to the sense of mineness of his experience, and hence, upon reflection, to a concern with self. At the same time, this same sense of his experience as changing through his experiencing of it is related to the sense of the moment as unshared, as mine only. This aspect of the lived moment, upon reflection, gives salience to the theme of interpersonal distance, which then is also a part of the I's reflected experience. The two themes are connected by way of the I's sense of his experience as mediated.

Reflected Experience

Reflected experience as transforming course

What is peculiarly introverted in the I's reflected experience? There are two aspects of experience here that distinguish the experience of the I from that of the E. Both we shall fit eventually to Jung's dynamic model of introversion.

Let us review here the distinction between lived and reflected experience and add to it a bit. As noted earlier, the difference is that the latter is disengaged. Reflected experience is holding the world at arm's length. In holding the world at arm's length, there is awareness of the self as distinct from the world and yet related to it. The subject/object split is reinstated.

It is a characteristic of reflected experience that during a reflected moment one "arrest(s) the fleeting from the continuum of confrontations with the world" (Straus, 1966, p. 70). In other words during a reflected moment, there is a fixing of the moment or happening within the context of one's other thoughts and feelings or vis-à-vis what one has had of other contacts in the world. By so fixing the moment, it is taken in its relation to one's self. In the lived moment, however, since the self is "forgotten" in the being absorbed in the moment, this self-reflection is precluded. While self-reflection cannot be part of lived experience, it is a necessary part of reflected experience.

To illustrate let us return to an earlier example. You are having a heated discussion in which you become absorbed and forget yourself. This is a lived experience. But then from time to time you step back and think about the thoughts or more broadly the experience you were having in the discussion. This moment in which you step back and make an object of what you were experiencing is reflected experience. In fact you probably reflect on what you were experiencing as a function of how important it was to you and these reflections may occur periodically for a long time afterward.

Now here we are approaching not so much a characteristic of reflected experience per se as a statement of the relation between reflected experience and the lived moment. In doing so we are simplifying that relationship. In the above example, it was presumed that the reflected moment is only a reflection on an earlier lived moment. In fact, the relationship is much more complex and interactive. We have simplified it since we are interested only in developing some characteristics peculiar to the I's view of his reflected experience. A strikingly clear experiential description of this relationship in its actual complexity is contained in Gendlin's *Experiencing and the Creation of Meaning* (1962). Part of his thesis is that reflection gives explicit meaning to the implicit "felt-meanings" which constitute lived experience. He further maintains, however, that the act of reflecting also "advances" meaning. Meaning, in part, is "created" in this way.

For the purpose of describing the I's reflected experience, we shall employ the term "assimilate" instead of "advance." While the sense of reflected activity as advancing felt-meanings is experientially more accurate, the term "assimilate," and the idea that reflected experience involves an assimilative function for the individual, provides a better basis for what is to follow. We introduce it explicitly as a conceptual tool, an aid to theorizing about the function of reflected experience. The theory states that the function of reflected experience is to assimilate and to store the stuff of one's contacts in-the-world, the stuff of lived moments. Once we have employed this notion as a temporary scaffolding, the present aspect of the I's reflected experience will stand on its own.

To return to our example, as you reflect on what you took from or had during the discussion an assimilative process is going on. The stuff of your lived experience, the thoughts and feelings, are being shaped and molded, fitted into existing schemes, put into a memory storage, or the like. We would assert that the I and E have different views of this assimilative process of reflected experience. They have different views of their reflected activity.

The *I* perceives the assimilating process as one in which the original thoughts and feelings which he took away from the discussion are transformed. His experience of his reflected activity accentuates transformations of his thoughts and feelings in the course of his reflection. More precisely, he senses that through his reflection on them, they are being transformed. Because they are seen as being transformed, reflected activity is sensed as having a course or path. The perceived course becomes an object of focus which he observes and notes in its growing and changing. This organic process is then sensed as having its own "life." This present feature of the *I*'s reflected experience is of a piece with and so complements his sense of the lived moment as mediated—as changed. In the lived moment, the latter is a given part of his experience, a sense of what he is experiencing as being changed. His view of his reflected activity as a transforming course is a complementary experience of a process of mediation itself. The immediately given sense of changing is viewed in reflection as a process, in particular as a transforming process.

The *E*, on the other hand, views the assimilating process of reflected activity less as transforming and more as an integrating, or a reorganizing of the original thoughts and feelings. It is perceived primarily as a recording of the thoughts and feelings given in the lived moment. In being assimilated, they are not seen as changing in any essential way. This view of his reflected activity as assimilative only in the sense of a recording and a reorganization is consistent with his sense of the lived moment as presentative or directly given, as more directly the encounter itself. He views his reflected activity as a process involving presentativeness. His thoughts and feelings are, to him, recordings or mirrors.

An analogy from photography may serve to clarify the distinction. The assimilating process for the *E* is like the process of developing a picture. While he may crop or highlight certain elements in the process of development, the *E* is always focused on the fact that he is working with a reflection of an object in the world. For the *I*, a new product is being made out of the stuff of his contact in the world. A raw stuff is being transformed into a new product; it is radically changed.

Reflected experience as becoming self

We have said that for the *I* the course of his thoughts and feelings in reflection is itself an object. It is viewed not only as a focal object but as an object of fascination, the basis of which lies in the recognition that the thoughts and feelings are being transformed, that they are growing and changing, and that they have a rich and intricate course. In this course they are not simply recorded and reorganized, but almost magically changed. The quality of transformation implies a quality of emergence. Something is being changed into something else. There is the unpredicted appearance of new characteristics in the course of reflected activity which underlies his fascination with it.

There is, however, an additional and most important reason why this life of his thoughts and feelings is an object of fascination to the *I*. The thoughts and feelings in their course are viewed as his *becoming self*. What is sensed as transformed, as emergent, is the self, that which will be viewed by the *I* as himself.

Let us explicate this idea by beginning with a truism that "we are our experience." If in reflecting itself an individual sees himself changing, he will store as his experience the sense that reflection itself is fascinating because it is a movement toward the emerging self. The *I* is fascinated with the course of his thoughts and feelings in reflection because he views that course as his becoming self. He senses each change as a change toward the form, substance, and particularity that will constitute his self, or what he will view as his self.

To emphasize this peculiarly introverted aspect of reflected experience let us contrast it with that of the *E*. How is it different for him? Are his thoughts and feelings in reflected experience not assimilating and storing the stuff of his contacts in-the-world? Are they not seen as becoming a part of self? Yes, they are, but only in that they are being recorded and reorganized through his reflected activity. They do not have the transformed quality that the *I*'s thoughts and feelings have for him. They are viewed simply as being transported by way of his reflected activity.

Accuracy is the salient dimension in the *E*'s view of his reflected activity. The validity question is important for him. Does he mirror the moment in what he eventually stores? Is what he eventually has of the moment the same as the moment? His concern with the accuracy of portrayal of his contacts in-the-world constitutes an overriding aspect of his reflected experience. With this view of his reflected activity, it is clear that the original contact and the thoughts and feelings directly born of the contact remain the locus of fascination for the *E*. It is as if the *E*'s main concern is to "have the world as it is"; while the *I*'s main concern is to "have his own world." The *E*'s reflected activity does not have the transforming, the magical, or the emergent quality, and hence the fascination that it does for the *I*. The truism that the *E* is a product of his experience still obtains. But what he comes to view as self is more directly the peculiar path of his contacts in-the-world and not some transforming course of his own reflected activity.

We need to add two qualifications to this description of the *I*'s "reflected experience." First, we do not mean to imply that the *I* displays a peculiar cognitive style in reflected experience. Although we employed a theoretical scaffolding along the way, the terms of which were cognitive ("assimilation," "storage"), what we are describing is an aspect of experience, an overriding sense or view of reflected experience which has its basis in Jung's dynamic model of introversion and our work with the TAT.

Second, in pointing to the *I*'s greater fascination with his reflected experience, we are not saying that he ends up knowing more about his thoughts and feelings or those of others. There are "psychologically-minded" but extraverted individuals who are attuned to the nuances of thoughts and feelings from moment to moment.* Clearly, not all clinical psychologists are introverts. The distinction is that accompanying the introvert's awareness of the nuances of his thoughts and feelings is a focus on their course, a sense of the transforming nature of that course, and a sense of them as his becoming self.

Experiential referents: Reflected experience and the dynamic model

It was argued earlier that some features of the *I*'s lived experience provide experiential referents for Jung's structural model. Now we are ready to show how characteristics of the *I*'s reflected experience provide similarly for the energy model.

In chapter 1 we established that "turning inward of the libido," a phrase applied to introversion by Jung, could be understood in terms of an energy model implicit in his writings. In that model Jung conceives of introversion as a movement of energy in a particular

---

*A "psychologically-minded" person, according to the California Personality Inventory, is an individual who is sensitive to the thoughts, feelings, and actions of others from the point of view of the "motives" and "inner needs" that they imply (1964, p. 11).

direction from object to subject. Introversion is defined as the movement itself, not as some state arrived at once this movement is accomplished. How is this directional movement of energy experienced?

The movement has its experiential referent in the I's reflected sense that his thoughts and feelings have a course. They "move" in that they are perceived as changing or being transformed in time. Such an image implies a path, and the movement suggested in Jung's writings is the sensing of this path. In examining Jung's energy model we found that part of what is meant by subjective view is one's "own psychological processes." The subject, as person, and his own thoughts and feelings are almost equated in this model. In describing the experience of a subjective view, which is the I's view, we are following this lead.

The second part of the energy model, the directionality of movement, finds its experiential referent in the second aspect of reflected experience that we have described. Movement "inward" from object to subject is captured in the experiential fact that the I's thoughts and feelings in their course are sensed as his becoming self. The movement from object to subject is experienced reflectively as moving toward becoming himself.

For the E, the direction of movement from subject to object has its experiential referent in a sense of his thoughts and feelings moving toward an increasingly accurate and inclusive representation of his contacts in the world. We would postulate that his sense of self is founded and built on a direct knowing of the world, a direct knowing of the object.

In addition to ties with Jung's energy model, these salient characteristics of the I's reflected experience may be linked to some empirical results. We have said that the I focuses on the transforming course of his thoughts and feelings in reflected experience. Since what he eventually stores of his contacts in-the-world is seen as radically changed through his reflection on it, he arrives at a sense of a world that is unique, his only. He feels that his world, his experience, is his alone. Concordant with that is a sense of being *worlds apart* from the "other" interpersonally. He is apart from the other by virtue of the perceived transformed nature of his experience, by what he perceives as his peculiar rendering of the world. Within this experiential framework the theme of distance which we found variously expressed in the TATs of Is is more readily understandable.

The unshared aspect of the lived moment together with the transformed aspect of the reflected moment suggest a sense of interpersonal distance. The sense of being worlds apart from the other is the experience of the distance theme in the TATs of the *I*.

Another descriptive aspect of the peculiarly introverted view of reflected experience recalls the second main theme of the TAT project, that of self-concern. What is it in experience? The *I*'s self-concern is intimately related to his fascination with his reflected experience. Part of his self-concern is a focus on his reflected experience as his becoming self. The *I*'s self-concern in experience is not directly a focus on or a fascination with self or person. It is a fascination with what is sensed as an ongoing process contributing to an evolving or emergent self. This, at long last in experiential terms, is Jung's reference to the subjective view as "own psychological process" and as a movement of energy from object to subject.

In an earlier section under the heading "lived experience," we discussed the two empirically obtained themes, self-concern and distance, as they are related to the *I*'s sense of his lived experience "as-changed." We argued that the *I*'s sense of the moment as "mine," as changing through his experiencing of it, gave salience to the theme of self-concern, while his sense of the moment as unshared, as "mine only," gave salience to the theme of distance. In the present context the *I*'s view of reflected experience as a transforming course reveals both his fascination with the becoming self and his sense of being worlds apart from others. These are the experiential counterparts of the themes of self-concern and distance respectively. The experiential referents of the two themes from the analysis of fantasy productions of *I*s are related by this common view of reflected experience.

The Broader Contours: Views of Self

Introduction

At this point, we have completed that part of the description of the experience of the *I* which directly provides experiential referents for Jung's two models. Much of what follows builds on the aspects of lived and reflected experience already presented. Part of our purpose here is to exhibit these aspects in a different setting and clarify them further. We hope to demonstrate their centrality in understanding the world of the *I* by indicating their applicability to other parts of that world.

The remaining sections have been organized into a set of special topics which will round out our picture of the introvert. The topics may be thought of as proceeding from the *I*'s view of his "experience," to his views of self, to a posture of self vis-a-vis the world, and, finally, to the *I* with another person. The direction of flow is from the finer fabric of the *I*'s experience, with which we began, to the broader contours of that experience. In a way, also, there is some movement away from description from the experiential point of view to description from a vantage point external to the *I*'s experience as felt.

Active maker of "experience"

Let us consider another usage of the term "experience" in addition to lived and reflected experience. It is the term as it might be employed by the man in the street and refers to what a person means when he speaks of "his experience" or says "in my experience." Stated more completely, when a person takes a long and extensive look at where he has been in life, at what he has done, at all his contacts and encounters with the world and at all his thoughts and feelings about these contacts, he might refer to what he sees as his "experience." It is a sense of the sum of his contacts with the world, what he has of his own cumulative life history. To look at his "experience," or by the act of looking at it, a person makes of it a thing. His "experience" is a possible object of reflection and when the look occurs it does so in reflected experience.

Both *I*s and *E*s have characteristic views of "experience" considered in this sense. For the *E*, "experience" is viewed directly as the sum of the events, the encounters with people, the ideas, and the like, to which he was exposed. When the *E* refers to or thinks about some set of contacts with the world such as his years in grade school, or his relationship with a best friend, or his summer in Europe, his view is consistent with statements of the form: What I was exposed to in grade school . . .; what I saw (did) on my trip to Europe. . . . What he was exposed to is seen as directly constituting his stored experience, his "experience." A consequence and, at the same time, a part of this view is that he sees his "experience" as something of which he was or is the passive recipient. He is the collector or storer of the stuff of his contacts. He has acted on it through his organizational efforts and through his checks on its validity, through his concern with whether what he has of it records accurately what it is. These acts, however, are not perceived as formative; the character of that which is stored is seen as resting in the contact itself.

For the *I*, that which he eventually has of a contact, that which he takes from the contact, or what is the contact for him is felt to be largely determined by the fact that he was a party to it. When the *I* refers to some set of contacts with the world, he is more apt to make statements of the form: What I "got" out of grade school . . .; what impressed me about my trip to Europe. . . . For the *I* what he was exposed to does not constitute his "experience"; rather, it is what he made or makes of the exposure. My fourth grade teacher, Miss Riley, is not my teacher, my "having" of Miss Riley is my teacher. This view is, of course, a derivative both of the mediated aspect of his lived moment, his sense of it as "my rendering," and of his view that the stuff of his contacts is changed or transformed as he reflects on it.

For the *I*, then, his "experience" is something of which he senses that he is the responsible author or the active maker. He senses that he is the primary formative agent of his "experience."

From this point, another follows directly. Each individual, whether an *I* or an *E*, thinks of the sum of his contacts with the world as *his* "experience." Everyone has a sense of "my experience." But for the *I*, the possessive has a more laden meaning and a more central thrust. He feels he is its active maker. This emphasis on the mineness of his "experience" is an extension of the given sense of mineness in the lived moment. Again, we have arrived at the saliency of the possessive in the *I*'s world.

Felt-substantiality of "experience"

The introverted way of sensing "experience" tends to make it more of a distinct and separate thing. For the *E* "experience" is also a thing and an occasional object of reflection. But considered as such it is more likely perceived by him as equated with the environment of his past, his background, the situations and things and people to which he was exposed, the things that he did. The events of his life are themselves his "experience." His "experience" is synonymous with the events that were their occasion.

For the *I* the event and his "experience" of it are sensed as two more or less distinct things. For him to say what his "experience" was is quite distinct from describing the event or the contact with the world itself. The *I*'s sense of his "experience" is reified in a way which is distinguishable from that of the *E*. The *E* makes a thing of his particular path in the world, the events in time and space in which he has participated. For the *I*, "experience" itself is a thing which is clearly very much other than the events which occasioned "experience." This view of its distinctiveness gives his "experience" a felt-substantiality. It is substantial in that it points less directly to the contacts of which it was born. It is less transparent, thicker, and has a kind of density and opacity.

These views of his "experience," and particularly of felt-substantiality have important interpersonal implications and concomitants. We shall develop these further in a later section describing the *I* with another. For the present let it suffice to reiterate that the *I* views his "experience" as his own, distinct from the events or exposures during which it was born. It is a focus of interest and fascination for him, a central part of his world.

Locus of definition of self

We turn now to what constitutes a peculiarly introverted view of self. Our earlier discussion of the *I*'s view of reflected experience as his becoming self provides a principal direction for the description.

The first aspect to be considered is the perceived locus of definition of self. This is to be distinguished from a more familiar topic, locus of self. The question is not where is the self or where am "I" located? It is, rather, where or what do I perceive as the "growing point" of self? at what interface is the self defined and constituted?

Let us begin with the *E*, who more than the *I* defines himself directly by his contacts in the world. From his view of reflected experience as a record or a more organized copy of his particular path of contacts in the world, the *E* perceives self in light of that path. He is constituted, in his view, by what he does, where he goes, whom he meets. His definition of self has as its perceived locus the set of those contacts. His "experience" and the self are perceived as identical with the particularity of his path through the world. Again, he is constituted by that path; it is the interface at which he perceives his self defined and redefined through time.

Turning to the *I*, he senses his work or his part in what he eventually "has" of his contacts in the world. The locus of this work is the perceived transforming course of his thoughts and feelings in reflection. Since this reflected activity is sensed as moving toward what will constitute self, the perceived locus of definition of self is the interface of his reflected experience and his becoming self. But now the experiential description is dangerously close to an objectified, conceptual framework and the experiential referents in the description may be slipping out of view. What is the *I*'s felt-locus of definition of self? It is simply a sense that there is a continual *self-definition of self*. The perceived locus of definition of self, in the world of the *I*, is the self.

This descriptive statement from any logical or philosophical point of view is a problematic if not impossible one. It is hopelessly (or perhaps delightfully) circular. Experientially, however, it is clear; and it is an ineluctable extension of the descriptive formulation to this point. The statement also provides further experiential formulation of Jung's association of the "subject" (here self) with "psychological process" (here reflected activity) which we puzzled over in chapter 1.

This difference in locus of definition of self has immediate implications for an aspect of control related to the self. An I/E difference here as elsewhere does not involve a difference in actual degree of control but in how control is perceived. Let us turn to a comparison between *I* and *E* on this issue. What is the meaning or context of this felt-control over who I am or who I define as self?

The question of control arises for the *E* in relation to what he has been able to accomplish and the what or whom of his contacts and encounters. To the extent that he can control the path of his contacts, the *E* feels that he controls what he is and will become. The *E* with a high degree of perceived control feels he can pick and choose the kinds of "experiences" he has in the world. A high degree of perceived control also implies a kind of activism that is peculiarly extraverted. It is a view of the world as manipulable and of the self as its effective manipulator. An *E* with less perceived control of locus of definition of self is apt to view the particulars of his path through the world as governed by chance, fate, or conspiracy.

The *I*'s sense of control is a function of his view that he is the responsible maker of his "experience." His "experience" originates in his rendering or his retelling of the moment and in his authorship of its transformation in reflected experience. Consistent with these perceived origins the I's sense of control emerges from his activity on that which he will perceive as his "experience" and that which he will perceive as his self. The activity gives his contacts in the world their character. Thus activism for the I with a high degree of perceived control of definition of self involves a sensed control of the reworking of what the world offers. It does not involve, as it does for the E, direct control over or direct manipulation of the particulars of what the world is to give and of what the self is to be.

The I with less perceived control senses the rendering in the moment or the transformation in reflection as intrusive. The possessive loses its salience for him. That the thoughts and feelings are a rendering is still part of his experience, but it is no longer his rendering. The thoughts and feelings are sensed as thrust upon him. No longer the possessor, he is possessed. This sense of intrusiveness is taken directly from Jung's theory and description of neurosis and applied to the present context (for example, see 1953, p. 237).

Self as unique

The I's sense of his reflected experience as his becoming self has led us to propose an I/E difference in locus of definition of self. A second postulated descriptive characteristic, the I's sense of his reflected experience as transforming course, leads us to consider an I/E difference in perceived uniqueness of self. Let us compare the world of the I and the E in this regard.

If he accentuates the uniqueness of self, the E grounds it in the particular path of his contacts with the world. Since his self is seen as comprised more directly of this set of contacts and of the thoughts and feelings to which they give rise, the degree of perceived particularity of the set determines the strength or accentuation of a sense of uniqueness of self. The E's view might be made explicit in the following form: I took my degree at W University, interned at X Hospital, worked with Dr. Y and did a paper on Z. I am sure no one else has taken quite this route, hence I am unique.

The I's sense of the uniqueness of self, as we have already suggested, is a derivative of his view of his reflected experience. The perceived transforming course of his thoughts and feelings in reflection together with the sense of them as his becoming self provide the ground for uniqueness. The I's feeling might be of the form: My thinking (feeling, etc.) about the event has had a fairly intricate course. Surely, it could not be duplicated in another person, hence I am unique. The perceived intricacies of his reflected activity yield the sense of uniqueness of self. It is not the different places he has been or things he has done; it is what he has gotten out of or made of those contacts which is the ground of his felt-uniqueness.

Beyond this initial grounding, the introverted sense of uniqueness is reinforced in a second way which makes the process a circular one from an "objective" point of view. The *I* perceives himself as the responsible maker of his "experience" and as the self-definer of self. This is to say that as the thoughts and feelings become evident, this unique self is seen as molding them. The thoughts and feelings are seen as changing, by virtue of their approach toward a presently perceived unique self, toward that very feature of uniqueness. More simply, a person perceiving himself as unique renders uniquely in his view, and perceives his consequent growth as movement along a unique line.

In addition to this difference in the form or the grounding of a sense of uniqueness of self, there is an I/E difference in the prominence or salience of uniqueness. To describe this difference we return to the description of the lived moment. For the *E*, there is a sense of the sharedness of what he is given in the moment. Remember the *E*'s focus on the sameness of the sights in the mountain clearing of our earlier description. By extension, a sense of sharedness, of commonality with the other is prominent. The *E* is feeling, to use a fresh example, that his classmates in the same graduate program are having the same experiences as he is; or at least, he is emphasizing the sharedness or sameness of that experience. The *I*, on the other hand is focused on the mediated nature of his experience in the moment. What he is experiencing in the engaging moments in the classroom or in discussion is sensed as changing through his experiencing of it. It is his rendering or version. Further, a concomitant of this emphasis on the mediated aspect of the moment is that it is sensed as his only. What he is experiencing is sensed as different from that which his classmates are experiencing, and hence unique.

The path that we have followed in our description, from lived to reflected experience, to view of "experience," and, finally, to view of self, suggests the prominence for the *I* of the view of self as uniquely constituted, in counter-distinction to the *E*'s emphasis on a sense of sharedness, of commonality of self with others.

Self as emergent

Still another source of difference in view of self involves attitudes toward the growth or development of self. The E views the growth of self in terms of the path of his contacts through the world. As he does more, sees more, comes in contact with more, the self is seen as developing by being built on wider swaths or more extensive samples of the world. The broader swath is for him an increasingly accurate and comprehensive knowing of the world. This sense of increasing knowledge of the world constitutes the perceived growth of self. In the E's view his cumulative journey through the world is inseparable from the growth of self. The self is developing in that there is a sense that it is being constituted by larger and larger segments of the world.

The emphasis in this perception of self-development is not on the self per se. It is on the world upon which the self is being founded. In particular it is on the accuracy and inclusiveness of the increasingly known world. The E sees himself growing as he knows more of the world. Paralleling an earlier point about the E's view of his "experience," the self is seen as less separate an entity than is the case for the I. We do not mean that there is confusion in boundaries between self and world. The point is that the E's view emphasizes a self made of the very same stuff that is the world or his contacts with the world. As such there is less emphasis not on self as a separate entity, but on self as *sui generis*, as a peculiar or unique class of things in the world. This is distinct from and must be added to the earlier point that there is less emphasis by the E on his particular self as unique among other selves. The perceived movement of self is toward more extensive shared ground, toward greater commonality with other selves.

One final point in the E's view of self is that growth occurs by a process of continual summation. The path of contacts through the world becomes more crisscrossed in a tighter weave. Growth is cumulative and its focus is the path of contacts, and the accuracy with which the world is both immediately experienced and later reflected.

The introverted view of growth of self is in striking contrast to that of the E. As we have described, the I's view of self is intimately related to the perceived transforming course of his reflected activity.

In the present context, this descriptive phrase can be expanded and recast. The *I* views the growth of self as "emergent" or "transcendent." These terms refer to the *I*'s sense that the self is something other than the stuff of which I was and am being made. It is other than the path of engaged moments in the world because it is sensed as changed in the moment; it is other than the assimilated thoughts and feelings in reflection because these are sensed as radically changed, as transformed.

The theme of emergence is central in Jung's explorations of the "collective unconscious" (see, for example, 1969, pp. 149ff). This is no accident, when we consider the relationship between introversion and the collective unconscious in his theoretical scheme. In the myths, folktales, and religious writings of various cultures investigated by Jung and his followers, emergence is portrayed graphically by the related themes of metamorphosis and rebirth. In this literature the self grows by being born again in successive and novel guises. Emergence is symbolically depicted through actual radical change, through a new life dramatically different from that from which it arises.

In terms of the present description, the self of the *I* is seen as emergent in the following sense: It is an entity being "born again," repeatedly, of the stuff of one's contacts in the world, which are seen as radically changed through the act of one's "having" of them. It follows from this that the *I* perceives the self as an entity *sui generis*. It is a peculiar "thing" unlike any other class or kind of thing. It also follows from this that the course of growth of self is perceived as saltatory, as proceeding by leaps. Radical change or transformation necessarily implies this.

With these points we are describing the basis in experience of the *I*'s "self-concern," a theme found empirically in the TATs of *I*s. We are also describing what constitutes the experience of that self-concern, the peculiarly introverted experience of self. From this description it should be immediately clear why, although everyone is to some extent interested or fascinated with self, the *I*'s world largely consists of themes which may be more accurately abstracted as self-concern.

For the *I* the self is sensed as unique vis-a-vis other selves; and the definition of self is located more in "introspective" or "reflective" activities than in the engaged moments which are the initial occasions for this work. The experience of reflected activity approaches a sense of on-going self-definition of self. The *I* in his experience does not directly have the world. He senses that his self is not founded directly in it. It is founded in his rendering of it.

Empirical and experiential ties

In chapter 2 we presented three rules related to the general theme of self-concern. At this point let us draw some connections between these rules and experiential aspects of self. One subtheme was an expressed comfort with the exclusive company of self and/or with "being with" one's own thoughts and feelings. These expressions of comfort may be linked to the introverted focus on and fascination with reflected activity and with the self seen as developing through emergence.

A second subtheme was the peculiarly introverted mode of resolving stress by relying upon the self. This is in keeping with the *I*'s view of himself as the responsible maker of his own "experience," and his view of the transforming course of his reflected activity. His "experience" or his values or standards are seen as less directly given by others. They are perceived as a product of the fact of *his* experiencing them in the moment and in reflection. Hence when a situation occurs in which there is a choice between recourse to self and to others for an evaluation of a present negative feeling, the *I* is more likely to rely upon "internal" standards or his own past experience for solution.

But why is this recourse to self not more generally descriptive of the *I*? Or in interpersonal terms, is it not introverted to be generally disaffiliative and aloof from others? We have failed to find evidence both in an experiment and in thematic material that this is the case. The *I* is less affiliative than the *E* only in a particular and circumscribed set of situations and not in all situations. The third subtheme within the theme of self-concern will help us to describe in experiential terms how direct recourse to self and turning away from others are not generally characteristic of the *I*. At the same time we shall move from views of self to the broader scope of the self/world relation

Self in relation to the world: World as stimulator

Reflected experience, as distinct from lived experience, takes "being" out of the world and makes of the world an object separable from the subject. That it does so necessarily implies a particular posture by the person to the world. The way in which a person objectifies indicates a particular orientation or attitude toward the world. This way of approaching the world is an aspect of experience that is felt at some level virtually every moment.*

For example, the world may be seen as a place which one tries to make better, a thing to try to improve. Or an "engineer" may approach the world as a set of material to be harnessed or manipulated toward more expedient or efficient ends. Or a "scientist" may approach the world as an object which is to be understood by "neutral" observation from a position conceptualized as external to it. These postures are felt-relations between the world in its totality as an object and one's self also as an object in a particular position in regard to it.

For the *I* the world is a place which provides raw material for the stimulation of his thoughts and feelings. A clear example is contained in the third subtheme of self-concern (Rule 1, card 1), which dealt with the boy and the object usually perceived as a violin. In the stories of introverts the boy is more likely to approach the violin as an object of fascination to wonder and puzzle about than as a means of achieving fame or fortune. This story is an explicit thematic expression of the introverted posture.

A second example of this introverted posture is taken from Jung's autobiographical account, *Memories, Dreams, Reflections* (1965), although it is not labelled as such there. The setting is his childhood home at a time when his father is on his deathbed:

> There was a rattling in his throat, and I could see that he was in the death agony. I stood by his bed, fascinated. I had never seen anyone die before. [p. 96]

In this otherwise grievous and traumatic moment, at least a part of Jung's experience is that the world is offering him stimulation. An event novel to him is occurring before his eyes. His posture to the event or in the event is that here is indeed food for thought. Here is a contact with the world through which he will have "new" thoughts and feelings.

In this peculiarly introverted relation to the world, the world is perceived as the necessary stimulator. It is not seen merely as a stimulator which functions as a triggering device; nor is it seen

---

*In Merleau-Ponty's term, it is felt horizontally (1962, p. 68).

merely as an initiator or an occasion for a thought or feeling. In reflection this posture includes a sense of the intimacy required in the self-world interaction. To be stimulated the *I* must become engaged or immersed in the world and forget his self in the lived moment. As we described, it is given as a sense of the mineness of his experience, and as a sense of his own part in what is his peculiar rendering of the moment. The *I*'s lived moment, so experienced, is the prime instance of this procurement of stimulation. In reflection, the *I* makes explicit the world as an object with this stimulating character, and his relation to it.

The point is that the world is as crucial to the introvert as it might be to a less introverted individual. As a particular posture to the world introversion implies continual approach and immersion. It is a stance in which a person confronts the world squarely and with some curiosity as exemplified in the encounter of the boy and the violin. The *I* obtains stimulation from the world by being in the world.

This posture is not consistent with a general tendency toward disaffiliative behavior; nor is it consistent with a generalized aloofness from the world. If the *I* did not immerse himself in the world he would lose the major potential source of his stimulation. Such a mode of being would be that of an unrealized *I*. It would be a mode of being most probably indicative of pathology.

This world-as-stimulator posture in part constitutes the *I*'s self-concern. It is a posture in which the *I* is "using" the world to stimulate his own thoughts and feelings. Eventually, through his reflected activity on these he will add to his "experience" and to that which is viewed as self. Thus the posture in part constitutes his self-concern and, from an external point of view, is simultaneously in the service of his self-concern. It provides the stuff for his reflected activity which is then perceived as his becoming self.

Thus we see that the *I*'s self-concern is a salient characteristic of aspects of his experience resulting from the peculiar way in which he is enmeshed in the world. It is not manifested as a focus on self in some contemplative, Buddha-like fashion, or perceived as encapsulated or cut off from the world.

If we examine these ideas in light of the TAT data we find that recourse to self in the sense of turning one's back on the world is a situationally limited response of the *I*. It is not at all indicative of his general posture to the world. When a situation presents an object or person of potential interest, an introvert no less than an extravert may approach and immerse himself in an encounter with that person or thing. When the situation is such that approach is not appropriate or demanded, it is introverted to be comfortable with the exclusive company of one's own thoughts and feelings. Finally, in a stressful situation, that general posture to the world or to objects in the world is disrupted and there is no approach. Under such conditions it is introverted to turn away from the world and from social comparisons to the self as the preferred locus of evaluation. Only under stress is the *I*, both from the points of view of his appearance to others and of his own experience, more like the popular picture of a disaffiliative, retiring individual. To hold this view more generally about the *I*, we believe, misses the mark in terms of a more fundamental understanding of introversion.

There is one further relationship we would like to draw in the attempt to tie together the description of the *I*'s posture with ideas elaborated earlier. The world-as-stimulator posture recalls a feature of the dynamic model discussed briefly in the first chapter. Jung stated that the "introverted attitude" is an "abstracting" one in that it involves drawing or taking away energy from the object. The present description of introversion appears consistent with that formulation. However, the Jungian notion of abstraction as presented within the energy model of introversion may be misleading in at least one important aspect when applied to the world of the *I* as experienced. Jung's terminology emphasizes the world as an object which the *I* depletes through abstracting. "Thus, for me, abstraction has the meaning of an energic *depreciation* of the object" (1933, p. 522, his emphasis).*

This notion of the world as an object from which one takes something is not supported by our empirical data. Abstraction as taking from or depleting suggests the operation of "using," or exploiting, which we reported in chapter 2. Our findings are equivocal when comparing *I* and *E* protocols containing this theme (Appendix

*Jung discussed at least two other usages of the term "abstracting." One is abstracting as taking from individual things their general similarities (1933, p. 64). This is akin to abstracting as concept-formation and brings to mind K. Goldstein's distinction abstract/concrete. Jung, however, explicitly distinguishes this first usage from the introverted attitude (p. 522). A second usage he borrows from Worringer (Jung, 1933, pp. 358–371). Abstraction is a removal of oneself from the object's influence. The object has an "operating force" whose influence a person may dread and from which a person defines himself by withdrawing from it (p. 362). We are not clear to what degree Jung associates this second usage with introversion. That it is not foreign in his thinking about introversion is evident from "On the Psychology of the Unconscious" (1953, p. 66).

B, p. 166). Further, this notion is not consistent with our experiential description which is based on more central features of both models of introversion. We do not think that the *I*'s felt-posture to the world includes a perception of the world as an object to be drained for his own gain. While the world is a place from which he "takes" stimulation, it is not part of the experience of the *I* that the world loses anything in the transaction. The felt-posture includes no sense of being an exploiter or stealer partly because he modifies what he takes. The "world-as-stimulator," not the "taking away from," is constitutive of the felt-posture.

Perhaps our difference with this aspect of Jung's conception of introversion can be reconciled by postulating variation in the experience of introversion. In particular, we need to consider pathological variations of the common introverted experience. This path is suggested since Jung was primarily involved with a clinical population and his thinking about introversion undoubtedly was influenced by this experience, despite his concern with rescuing introversion from any pathological tinges. Let us examine this matter in further detail.

While the introverted posture is not focally one of depleting the world, the *I* seeks stimulation of his own thoughts and feelings, which in reflection are viewed as his becoming self. As such the stimulation sought from the world is a form of self-stimulation. Further, although in the lived moment what is given is sensed unequivocally as mine, in reflection there may be some doubt as to the legitimacy of that sense of mineness, especially if the source of the stimulation is the words of another. Since the *I*'s posture to the world is one of receiving from it, and since the sense of ownership which is inherently ambiguous* is a central one for the *I*, the introverted experience is fraught with pathological possibilities. We hasten to add that in this regard it is different from any other approach to the world only in particulars, not in degree.

For the *I* there is the neurotic possibility of guilt associated with exploitation and egotism. In a different sector of the pathological spectrum, there is the possibility also that this posture can sustain a psychopathic adjustment. The *I* may come to view the world, like the psychopath, as a place where one must take what he can get and "devil take the hind-most."

We reported data in chapter 2 which suggest that this latter

---

*"We are referring again to Straus's point about the ambiguous and enigmatic character of sensory experiencing.

adjustment, rather than a guilt-ridden one, may be the more common pathological adjustment of the *I*. Bieler (1966) found that *I*'s are significantly less intropunitive than *E*s; and we found in the TAT project a trend for *I*s to include less self-blame in fantasy. To the degree that *I*s are less prone to self-blame, a poor adjustment may be more common in a psychopathic than in a neurotic form.

Aside from these pathological possibilities of adjustment, the *I*'s posture generally sustains an enriched sense of his reflected experience based on a fruitful interaction with and in the world. To reiterate, while the *I*'s back is not to the world and while he is not apart from it, neither is the world the center of his being. The world for him is a rich source of potential stimulation of his thoughts and feelings, viewed and sensed in reflected and lived experience in the various ways we have described. These thoughts and feelings with their intimate relation to his sense of self are the central focus for the *I*.

If the world is an ocean and the *I* its explorer, then the fascinating things to be explored are not directly in the ocean but are in his examination of his "finds." And yet, in order to explore and in order eventually to enrich self, he must submerge himself in the ocean.

Thus we have revealed the crux of the *I*'s problem with people, to which we now turn more directly.

The Broader Contours: The Introvert with an "Other"

The introvert's "people problem"

One of the reasons an *I* approaches people is that he needs them. In common with his less introverted brethren he has for better or for worse a full set of people needs. Whatever is introverted about a person, whatever introversion is, does not preclude interest in the gratification of these needs nor success in the effort. The bulk of the TAT material and our study on introversion and affiliation both offer limited evidence in support of this view. In terms of measures such as "amount" of interaction, number of relations with others, and degree of affiliation, the difference between the *I* and the *E* is not particularly telling. The *I*'s world generally is as much a peopled world as is the world of the *E*.

In referring to the *I*'s "people problem," we do not mean to suggest that introversion is necessarily associated in any simple quantitative way with a dearth of human relationships. The *i* has a people problem only in that like everybody else he needs to be with people. The *I*'s people problem refers only to those aspects of his interpersonal relations which are unique to his introvertedness. What we need to describe is the form and the particular problems which the introverted experience and posture give to interpersonal relations, or, more generally, what it is like for an *I* to be with people. The question whether an *I*'s peculiar interpersonal experience makes his relations with others more or less difficult or gratifying than the less introverted individual is one we are not ready to confront. In fact, it would seem a moot question. If two people have the same biological needs but different ways of experiencing and approaching the world, who is to say if one enjoys what he is more than the other? We can only state that we assume an equivalence of need for people.

Being with a person or thing

We have described the *I*'s typical posture to the world. Now we shall add another dimension to that description. One way in which different postures to the world can vary is in the degree to which they distinguish between people and things as objects. Within this framework they can vary further in the degree to which they give centrality or "specialness" to one or the other category. For example, if one's posture to the world is that it is a place upon which to make an impression or to have a remembered impact, then people as objects are both central and special, since only they are clearly and permanently impressionable. Similarly, if the world is a place in which to make oneself understood, then again people are central and special since only they have this capacity of understanding. Conversely, if the world is a place which arouses certain affects that one is concerned to avoid, then people are kept out of the center since they often arouse the threatening affects. In this case things might be more central since they are more congenial, less threatening. However, if the world is a place with which to have communion or to "be one with," then more often than not no distinction is made between person and thing. In this same vein if the world is a place which is to be understood, then probably no distinction will be made.

Finally, if the world is a place, as it is for the *I*, from which one obtains stimulation of one's own thoughts and feelings, stimulation intimately related to one's evolving or growing self, then there is no necessary distinction; nor is there any centrality or specialness given to the one class of object over the other. For the *I* an unpeopled situation can be as stimulating, in the particular sense in which we have been employing this term, as a situation in which another person is the focal object. A book or lecture, a mountain scene, a violin, or another person can be equally and adequately stimulating. Hence, on card 1 of the TAT, as we reported in chapter 2, the *I* more often tells a story which deals primarily with the boy and the violin. The violin is sufficient stimulation for his thoughts and feelings. Further, both on this card and on the second one (card 3 BM) in which an individual and a thing are pictured, the *I* more often does not introduce a second person (Appendix A, Rules 2 and 4). He does not bring a second person into his story because his own posture to the world gives no centrality or specialness to a person over a thing. On the other hand, given TAT cards with two people pictured as the central objects he is as likely as the *E* to see them as related or to see the relationship as the central stimulating object. Both people and things are potentially stimulating and no central or special importance is given to the one over the other.

We have already emphasized that the *I*'s posture does not preclude being engaged with the object and that the fruits of this moment are, upon later reflection, a major source of stimulation. Now we can add that the qualities given to the *I* in a lived moment are the same whether the object encountered is a thing or a person. Whether the *I* has an encounter with a book, a mountain scene, a violin or a person, what is experienced in that encounter is sensed as a rendering that is peculiarly his own.

This lack of obvious object preference may seem puzzling to those whose stance clearly includes such a preference. The *I* seems as readily engaged by and as comfortable with his own company and the company of nonpeopled settings as he does in social settings. On balance then the social setting would appear to be less preferred. It is this perceived devaluing that induces the popular notion of the *I* as aloof or schizoid. A closer look will produce the observation that the *I* is frequently engaged and stimulated in his own way by a meeting with another person.

The interpersonal paradox or reversal

This brings us to a paradox which is central to our description of the *I* with others. It is a paradox in the sense that it is something contrary to expectation. It involves a reversal or switching, in the I's interaction, of some qualities usually associated with the encounter or lived moment with some aspects usually associated with the reflected moment.

We usually think of an encounter as involving a baring of souls, or as a more or less successful attempt at an open sharing of views, or as an experience which is mutually shared. We speak of the relative authenticity of the encounter by referring to the degree to which what is shared is genuine and open for both parties. But, as we described earlier, for the I the encounter includes absorption in what is not sensed as a shared exchange. It is unshared because what is given to him in the moment is sensed as changing in his experiencing of it, as his peculiar version of the moment. The I's encounter is sensed as a private dialogue, a dialogue that is exclusively mine. With reflection the stuff of the dialogue is sensed as further transformed. This enhances his sense of the privateness of what he had of the meeting.

From the point of view of the other in the dialogue, the I again presents a puzzling combination of features. He seems a bit self-serving and a bit isolated in his own world. Yet upon closer examination he clearly seems to be engaged in the moment and fascinated with what is being discussed. Is he simply being manipulative and exploiting the situation to his own ends or interest? Is he self-serving, or is he genuinely enthralled by the topic and the moment itself? Or is there a distinction for him?

In addition to sensed mutuality a second characteristic usually associated with the experience of an encounter with a person is a reinforcement of the importance of the other person. This usually follows the encounter, after the subject-object split is reinstated. By this we do not mean simply an elevation of the specific other of the encounter but rather of other persons in general. The other is elevated because the relation and the sharing that constitutes the encounter is only possible with another person. Only we, two people, can have this together. Hence the other is important and valued.

The elevation of the other person does not follow in the aftermath of the encounter for an I. The other is a necessary part of the encounter but he is not sharing in what he, the I, has of the moment; nor is he sharing in what is focal to the I in the moment. That which is focal and elating to the I, the given version or retelling, is not shared by the other and is differentiated from the relation of which the other is a part. The other is necessary but not focal and, of course, the other does not need to be a person.

To put this another way, if the focal part of the experience is not the contact with the other but an unshared rendering of it, then both the contact and the other are less important. Thus there is for the *I* in the aftermath of the lived moment a relative devaluing of the other, not an elevation of him. The devaluing is only relative however. The other is less valued than the retelling, which through its association with (or through its being sensed as) the *I*'s becoming self, is elevated. "Devalued" is employed here not in the sense of degraded but in the sense of not being of focal interest. The devaluing is implicit, not only in the focal unshared retelling, but in the *I*'s posture to the world which does not distinguish object-as-thing from object-as-person.

As part of the nature of the *I*'s relations with people we have pointed out that the usually shared and usually other-elevating encounter is a private dialogue for the *I* in which the other is not special or elevated. This description of the *I*'s encounter with the other, incidentally, further explicates Jung's energy model of introversion. It depicts more precisely and in less experientially thin terms what Jung meant by a "negative relation of subject to object" as a characteristic of introversion.

To complete the picture of the *I*'s interpersonal relations we turn to the reflected moment. We need to introduce another feature of the *I*'s reflected experience, namely, his view of his transformed thoughts and feelings as a product. Recall the peculiarly introverted reification of his "experience," as other than the occasions that induced it. This distinctiveness, in his view, gives to "experience" a thickness, a density, an opacity. There is no sense of it as a reproduction which is transparent since we can "see through" it to the original. It is, rather, a substantive thing, a product. It is a product of his reflection, an end-result of his reflected activity, of the work that he senses he does not only in reflection but also in the primary engaged moment. And, given the pervasive introverted sense of mineness, founded both in his view that the part he plays as the experiencer of what he experiences is formative and in his view that the stuff of his contacts in the world, his thoughts and feelings, is moving toward his emergent self, it is, to him, *my* product.

Viewed as such and valued as such, the *I* employs his products interpersonally as a kind of currency. They are brought into an interaction as "a thought (or feeling) that I have had," or "an experience that I want to tell you about." The form of the *I*'s statement, implicit or expressed, is not "Let me tell you about what happened yesterday"; it is rather, "Let me tell you about what was my experience of what happened yesterday." This is the interpersonal expression of his focus on the mediated nature of his experience.

When the *I* employs his products in this way, he is attempting to share an end-result of his own reflection. The result of a moment in which the other and the world is held at arm's length and taken in reference to one's self is brought into the interaction as a medium of exchange. Here, what is usually thought of as private or "personal" is made public and becomes the stuff of an interaction with another person. This ready public use of the private or personal is the second part of the reversal.

What we are referring to will perhaps be most easily recognized in those moments with another person in which he seems to be straddling the line between discretion and indiscretion, between what is mildly embarrassing and what is intimate and appropriately personal.

For the *I*, while a lived moment is sensed as unshared with the other, as private and exclusively mine, the thought or feeling evolved from his reflection of that moment is shared with the other. What is usually thought of as shared is felt to be unshared; while there is an attempt to share that which more typically remains unshared.

Product as "standing between"

What is the interpersonal effect of the *I*'s attempt to share? His focus on his reflected thoughts and feelings as his product "stands between" the *I* and the other in that it usually prevents the lived moment or encounter. That it does so follows from the *I*'s view of it. His emphasis on the product's exclusive mineness, and on it as part of his self, maintains the saliency of the mine/other's distinction. This makes the forgetting of self and the transcending of the self/other distinction essential to an encounter unlikely to be accomplished. Ironically, in attempting to be personal, the *I* diminishes the likelihood of an encounter. His view of the introduced thought or feeling as distinct, transformed, and mine keeps the interaction from becoming an engaged moment.

A related instance also typical of the *I*'s interaction with another involves the disruption of an already on-going lived moment. Let us say an *I* is engaged with another. What is given to the *I* in the moment is sensed as a rendering or retelling that is exclusively mine. To share it, he must point at the moment as it was given to him. This makes of the moment a thing, and, of course, a thing that is viewed as mine. The self/other split is thus reinstated and the being absorbed ended. We may think of the disruption of the lived moment being announced with a statement by the *I* of the form—"while we have been talking, I have had the impression (feeling, or experience) that. . . ." Again this, at least temporarily, destroys the lived moment.

We take it to be typical of the engaged interaction of an *I* with an other that there is a kind of in/out movement, as first the lived moment is disrupted, then regained only to be disrupted again. Let us reemphasize that what we have described here is the *I*'s peculiar problem with maintaining and with establishing an encounter, and we do not suggest that his difficulty is greater than that of a less introverted individual.

We have insisted that the *I* typically tries to share with the other either his retelling of the lived moment or the product of his reflected experience. The question arises of why he tries. We could simply assert that he does so for the same reason any person shares something with another—because it is human to do so. Beyond this, however, some reasons make sense for the *I* in particular. He tries to share his rendering in the lived moment because he is often elated in the moment, and the elation easily spills over. He tries to share the product of his reflection because it was born of a contact that stimulated his thoughts and feelings. He gets his kicks out of it, and he assumes that the other both wants to and is able to obtain similar kicks. It has been and is stimulating to him, surely it will also excite the other. Finally, he tries to share his product because it is important to him. It is a focal part of his world.

The sense of interpersonal distance

We have already pointed out some aspects of the *I*'s sense of distance from the other. One aspect is implicit in the introverted sense of the lived moment as "changed" and "exclusively mine." It is made explicit, however, only in reflected experience. Through an awareness of the transformed course of his thoughts and feelings in reflection the *I* arrives at a sense of being worlds apart from the other.

This sense of distance is most poignant during transactions with others. The attempted sharing of his world with the other underscores the felt-distance, for it is precisely this unshared world which separates the *I* from the other. When his introverted world, his product, disrupts the encounter, it is in the resulting disengaged moment that the felt-distance is acutely present.

In other disengaged or reflected moments in which the *I* is alone there is, as the empirical evidence presented in chapter 2 suggests (Appendix A, Rule 7), a comfort with his thoughts and feelings, with his reflected experience. There is in these moments of solitude the excitement of the transforming course of his reflected activity and the fascination with the self, perceived as it is by the *I* as continually emerging from this activity. But the reflected moment in an interpersonal context has a discomforting tension for the *I*. In these moments his world, his product, is not only dense and opaque but also a weight which keeps him from the other. His product has excited him and he desires to share it. Its opacity, however, derived from its sensed-mediated origins, precludes his doing so. In the interpersonal sphere, the *I*'s world is a burden which generally stands between himself and the other. That world is simultaneously important and exciting, *his*, him, to-be-shared, and a distance between him and the other.

We do not intend to confine the *I*'s sense of distance solely to the disengaged moment with the other. It is pervasive, no less than the sense of stimulation he gets from his engagement in the world, his sense of the moment as-changed, and his sense of mineness. It undoubtedly is felt horizonally at all moments. However, it is underscored by the fact of the other and the attempt to be with him.

This is as far as we can presently go in understanding the *I*'s experience of distance. However, there are a number of conclusions which may be unintentionally implied by the concept of distance to which we should like to turn our attention.

We noted in chapter 2 that the *I* is not uniquely motivated to gain or maintain distance from the other. He neither actively pushes the other away nor actively keeps himself from approaching the other. He is not aware that he has any greater feeling of distance from the other than people with little introversion. The relative difference is apparent only to the observer. The *I* does not, as a general rule, sense a greater distance between self and other than between any other two persons. While he feels that he is not close to the other he also feels that others are equally distant from each other.

We should like to comment briefly on our usage of the term "distance." Various recent works which take as their subject modern man describe him as severed or alienated from the world and from nature and as incapable of relating to others in any real sense. This description stems from a number of related diagnoses of the modern world as the age of technology, of hyperstimulation, of the bomb, of anxiety, of the loss of meaning, and the like. In these analyses the term "distant" is often employed as descriptive of modern man and equated with severed. The dimension we employ is one of degree of felt-distance/felt-closeness between self and other, not of separateness/unity. The opposite of distant is close, not fused or connected.

A related contemporary use of the term makes it more or less synonymous with schizoid. In his recent book *Love and Will* Rollo May (1969) describes the "schizoid world" of modern man as "a condition in which men and women find themselves experiencing a distance between themselves and the objects which used to excite their affection and their will" (p. 29). The emphasis in this usage, in addition to a sense of unrelatedness, of lack of communication and of commitment, is on a lack of feeling. To be distant is to be apathetic, to have no feeling (see also *The Borderline Syndrome*, Grinker, 1968). The schizoid or distant person, the description goes on, has little sense of self; he is empty, impoverished and apathetic. Our use of the term distance implies yet another and opposite vantage point from which it may be seen. We see the *I*'s sense of interpersonal distance as accompanied by a sense of being a unique individual, a self-defined and defining individual, a becoming or evolving individual; and, at the same time, an individual who is immersed in the world and enriched by that immersion.

Summary and beyond

The material of this section on the introvert with another was presented to provide a glimmering of the way in which the peculiarly introverted aspects of lived and reflected experience insert the *I* into the interpersonal sphere. The description emphasized how the sensed mediated nature of the *I*'s experience results in a reversal of what is generally public with what is private, a reversal of the to-be-shared with the unshared. The *I*'s encounter is a peculiarly private affair since it is felt to be unshared in the moment. Perhaps to compensate for this, the *I* attempts to share his private thought or feeling. However, this attempt, since it is asserted as his reflected product and as intimately related to his own self-development, has a disengaging effect. The thrusting of his self-development on the other stands between the *I* and the other. The feeling of exclusive possession and the density and opacity of the *I*'s transformed world, all founded in his focus on the mediated nature of his experience, makes his world a cumbersome burden in an interpersonal setting. He needs to share this world, and yet it is a difficult task. The sense of interpersonal distance remains omnipresent.

This introduction to the interpersonal world of the *I* raises as many questions as it answers. Before leaving the topic we shall comment briefly on one or two of them to further demonstrate the general applicability of our basic experiential formulation. Does the *I*'s product always stand between himself and the other? or, more generally, is there always a sense of being worlds apart from the other? A related question indicating our preferred approach would be: What is intimacy for the *I* as distinct from the *E*?

Intimacy like any other aspect of an individual's life is construed from the fabric of his world. In this sense it must be defined by him and judged achieved or not in these terms. For the *I*, a prerequisite for intimacy is a comfort with his sense of distance, of being worlds apart. Interpersonally this comfort is expressed through a respect for and an acknowledgment of the fact of the other's own world.* The *I* confirms the fact of the other's world existing independently of his and without threat to it. In this way the sensed distance is confronted and accepted, and becomes the foundation of the meeting of the two. Their acknowledgment of the separation of their worlds is the necessary basis upon which the potential union, their potential intimacy, is built.

The form which this acknowledgment takes interpersonally is a kind of empathy. While empathy may at first glance seem difficult for the *I* from all that we have said of the nature of his experience, yet it may be defined within the introverted world. For the *I*, empathy cannot be a direct experience of what the other is having in

---

*In this brief section we are only developing the possibility of intimacy for the *I* with another *I* and the *E* with another *E*.

the moment. For example, the statement, "I feel his sadness," or "I feel sad at his sadness," would do violence to the I's sense of the moment as peculiarly his rendering. But the I may be "empathic" in a more general context. Given his sense of the mineness of the moment for himself, he may sense the mineness of the other's moment and thus establish an empathic link between the two. He can empathize with the other's sense of peculiar rendering. This is prior to and other than having the particulars of that rendering. In turn, the I seeks recognition of the mineness of his own rendering of the moment and, by extension, of his own world from the other.

With this kind of sharing of the unshared, this mutually felt acknowledgment of the other's world-for-him, there is a framework for and a possibility of intimacy. For the I, intimacy is a relationship in which there has been movement toward the other's knowing one's own world, and, the converse, toward knowing the other's world. We say a moving toward because the goal is problematic and elusive. It is problematic because of the I's focus on the mediated nature of his experience. This focus introduces at every moment the ambiguity of whether one is knowing the other's world or one's own rendering of it. Intimacy is elusive because of the I's sense of the becoming quality of his self and his world. He cannot make known that which is only becoming. Achievement of intimacy is laborious because of its sensed transformed character, its intricacy, and its density and opacity.

This strain toward intimacy by the I, whatever its difficulties, has a typical form interpersonally. The I responds to the other's remark, first with confirmation of it as the other's and then with a remark giving his own rendering of it, that is giving what he experienced in the moment on the occasion of the other's remark: I see your particular way of looking at the matter but it seems to me that it also implies . . . .

We shall leave this aspect of the I's world unfinished except to contrast it with that of the E to demonstrate that intimacy is also a problem for him. Also, we want to suggest, tentatively, that the extent to which both the I and the E can be intimate is the degree to which they are no longer exclusively introverted and extraverted.

While for the I intimacy is a relationship based on a mutual awareness of the unique value of each other's own world, for the E to be intimate is to have the same world. Intimacy is a joint movement of two individuals toward knowing the same world. By "world" is meant for the E not one's own world in the over-determined sense of the possessive for the I. The to-be-known-together world for the E, rather, is the only veridical world. It is "reality" to be shared. Intimacy is the adding together of two paths through the world, perhaps two particular paths, but two paths which, in the E's view, can summate to a veridical having of the world. The barrier to intimacy in a relationship for the E is the view that the other's path through the world is inaccurately recorded, that it is a portrayal which is incongruent with his own record. This perceived incongruity would deprive the relationship of the required basis for intimacy. The having of the same world would be impossible.

To make the contrast explicit, there can be no summation of worlds for the I. To have as the center of intimacy a congruence of worlds would be to destroy the I's world which is, for him, an own world and a unique self.

Appendix A. Seven "I" Rules

Rule 1

Card 1: Object pictured ("violin") is itself seen as interesting or stimulating.

Interest expressed in the object's aesthetic properties—its appearance, sound, etc.

Interest expressed in the task associated with the object—the skill, complexity, etc. of playing the instrument.

Concern with *present* performance.

Examples:

. . . contemplating the *sheer mystery* of this instrument.
. . . wants to know every bit of this instrument.
. . . the little boy is wishing he could play the violin.
He wants to touch it, to pick it up, and try to play it.
. . . beautiful music; to make the violin sing . . .
. . . this young man is thoroughly fascinated with the instrument before it. He is deciding whether or not to pick it up and see what makes it tick.
. . . the boy is curious and goes to the table and examines it noting how it is put together and made.
. . . he's thinking how beautiful this instrument is—what beautiful sounds could come out of it.

Do not score "broken instrument" theme.

Rule 2

Card 1: Mention of only the figure pictured; no "other" person is brought into the story.

Rule 3

Card 3 BM: Negative affect is associated with the figure, and the figure reacts in a self-reliant way—actively attempts to resolve the difficulty by recourse to self.

Examples:

. . . she is worrying about dreadful things . . . she will get up, take an aspirin, turn on the phonograph to force her mind off her troubles, go to bed early, and feel fine in the morning.
The boy has just dropped her and she thinks that life is finished.
. . . She soon outgrows this trite stage and finds other boys.

162

This is a boy, exhausted and totally discouraged, leaning on a bench ... but he will eventually be physically and emotionally rested, will get up and begin to concentrate on the world.
... gets over grief and goes back to work.
... homesick boy picks himself up and, enthralled, reads *Huck Finn*.

Note: "negative affect" inferred from use of words such as sad, lonely, worried, depressed, crying; or from the situation or person described (lost husband and son in accident, engaged in a bad task, disturbed person).

Do not score when figure reacts in passive, nonconstructive way (e.g.: praying, enduring; will continue to hope; will die early).

Also *do not score* when the figure's reaction is to seek aid from others (e.g.: will be cured by doctors; parents will forgive her; he comes back to her; thanks to what his father showed him).

Rule 4

Card 3BM: Mention of only the figure pictured—no "other" person is brought into the story.

Rule 5

Card 9BM: Either (1) Negative view of the figures or their way of life;

Examples:

This is a white chain gang taking a rest during the noon break. These are all typical ex-convict types, bums, and winos ...
The men are migrant workers who have spent the night in the field of the farm belonging to the parents of the boy in the picture. The men are embittered that their life is so hard ...
Work in this summer was slow for the transient fruitpickers because of the severe frosts earlier that spring. Everywhere you went looking for a job, there were ten others ahead of you in the same situation ...

Note: "negative" refers to the difficulty, hardship, reward, etc. associated with figures or their way of life. It does not refer to the implied feelings of the subject toward the figures. In the example above, the portrayal of the hard life of migrant workers is scored although the subject seems sympathetic toward them in their plight.

or (2) Emphasis on the unpleasantness of the context.

Examples:

> . . . these men have been stuck in this fox hole for a whole day . . .
>
> This is a traveling work crew in a rural area. They have come into this area late at night and are extremely tired. Not having any place particular to go, they collapse . . .
>
> These are soldiers during the lull of a battle . . . Some are asleep, some have dropped from exhaustion, some are thinking thoughts of terror that I expect people think during the war . . .

Note: Score for unpleasant context even if present moment not unpleasant. For example, a work/rest theme is scored if emphasis is on work situation as unpleasant although at the moment the workers are described as resting.

Judgment as to unpleasantness is required. For example, war setting is not necessarily unpleasant, as a victory party following a successfully waged battle.

Rule 6

Card 9BM: Significant distinction made between any one or more of the figures.

(1) One figure within the group singled out as different or members of the group contrasted with each other; distinctions may be made by separation, distinction between any one or more of the figures in viewpoint, mood, personality, within group role, status.

Examples:

> Tramps have gathered from all over the world to elect a king. The man who will be selected as king of the tramps is shown here as he reclines upon his throne of human misery and squalor . . .
>
> . . . Men have just run off a great batch of moonshine. The boy in foreground is standing watch . . .
>
> These guys have been working hard . . . They immediately collapse, although one little fellow, the youngest of the group, doesn't want to sleep. He is thinking . . .

(2) One figure described as a nonmember of the group.

Examples:

> These soldiers are resting after a rough hike . . . The guy in front is a teen-ager who has left school to go to the dentist. He sees these men and . . .
>
> A boy wandering throughout the countryside early in the morning has encountered a group of hobos sleeping. He doesn't know who or what they are . . .

Do not score when significant distinction is made between figures pictured and others who are clearly not pictured (e.g., They are no longer fearing for their safety, for they are sure they have outdistanced their pursuers).

Rule 7

Card 14:   If figure is described without allusion to specific others and there is either (1) indication of a habit of or a comfort or pleasure in solitude

Examples:

>... in a mood to be alone with himself ...
>... often sits looking ...
>... pleasure in solitude ...
>... alone often ...

Do not score when "excuse" for solitude is emphasized (such as alone because of interpersonal problem or failing, because feeling depressed, or because need to study all night) or anything that indicates that solitude is an unusual rather than an habitual or comfortable activity.

or (2) an indication of an introspective or "thinking" person— allusion to habit of thinking; to quantity or quality of thoughts; to thinking about own attributes or abilities; to thinking about general "philosophical" themes.

Examples

>... long period of serious thought ...
>... myriad of thoughts ...
>... alone and knows his own powers and abilities ...
>... question all things ...
>... various thoughts run through his mind ...
>Omar has a mind; he is an artist ...
>... thinking how complex and fantastic life is ...

Do not score love of or appreciation of nature theme.

Appendix B. Definitions and Results of Personal Interaction Variables

We defined two measures of moving toward or "action-toward" which occur within a relation. The first scores evidence of a nurturant relation. Tag words include: console, help, comfort, reassure, and cheer up. A typical story describes husband and wife, lovers, or mother and son in a situation where one gives comfort to the other following some bad news—often news of a loss. Although Es give more instances than do Is in the first pool, the trend washes out in the validation (I = 12, E = 21 for 300 stories; p = .15. I = 18, E = 22 for 400 stories, p = NS).

Another operation within this same general category emphasizes a moving toward another that implies the existence of or the formation of a more symmetrical or mutual relation. Typically, stories involving engagement or nuptial plans or the reunion of a separated couple are scored. The themes scored are action-toward in the sense of marriage, reunion, return from a trip, invitations to join. Results are similar to the previous operation (I = 3, E = 11 for 300 stories; p = .06. I = 14, E = 24 for 400 stories; p = .15).

Several measures of "action-away" fail to turn up any significant I/E differences. Operations include scoring themes of a person leaving the other for any reason, explicit rejection of the other, and leaving the relation more or less permanently. Instances of the latter, one member of a relation abandoning the other, are scored for Is slightly more than for Es in both the first sample and validating sample. The trend is statistically nonsignificant (I = 13, E = 7 for 300 stories; p = .25. I = 18, E = 15 for 400 stories; p = NS).

Within the category "action-against," we defined a measure of aggression adapted from Purcell (in Murstein, 1965). Instances such as each of the following are counted: fighting, criminal assault, getting angry, criticizing, resisting, coercing, being negativistic, lying, dominating, or restraining someone. This measure does not require evidence of an ongoing relation within which one member aggresses against the other. There is no I/E difference here (I = 35, E = 30 for 300 stories; p = NS). A trend does emerge, however, when this measure of general aggressivity is restricted to aggression within a relation. The operation is defined as follows: Score criticism, disapproval, ridicule, anger, or aggression directed at a "related" person, or aggression against a third person which clearly grows out of a primary relation (the "jilted" or unfaithful theme). We defined two people as "related" if they are described as blood relatives, friends, or more than casually involved with each other. Is more often describe relations involving this operation of action against (I = 25, E = 12 for 300 stories; p = .06). In the cross-validation only the directionality is retained (I = 28, E = 21 for 400 stories; p = NS).

The results of a measure of aggression turned inward or internal punishment is consistent with the above. There is a trend for Es to include in their stories more instances of suicide, self-depreciation, remorse, and guilt (I = 10, E = 16 for 300 stories; p = NS. I = 7, E = 14 for 400 stories; p = .19). This suggests that *E*s are more likely to blame themselves than others and *I*s vice versa. Bieler's study of the relation between I/E and punitive styles is consistent with these findings (1966). Employing the M-B as a measure of I/E, a modification of the Rosenzweig as a measure of punitive style, and the Rotter Incomplete Sentence Test as a neuroticism moderator, Bieler found that *E*s are more intropunitive than are *I*s. This held for the whole population (N = 95, p = .02) and for low-neurotics only. A replication of this study by R. Ginsberg and the present senior author gave only a trend in the same direction. Pooling the data yielded a significant finding (N = 198; p = .04).

Two other measures which may be included in the category of action-against, broadly defined, are asymmetric relations and exploitative relations. We score a relation asymmetric when one of the members in the relation is described differentially as to dominance, worth, and the like. This is not scored for relations culturally prescribed as asymmetric such as employer/employee. Again, there is only a trend—*I*s are more likely than *E*s to describe a relation as asymmetric (I = 11, E = 4 for 300 stories; p = .12. I = 22, E = 15 for 400 stories; p = NS).

There is also a trend for *I*s more often than *E*s to view a relation in terms of one person exploiting or "using" the other (I = 13, E = 5 for 300 stories; p = .09. I = 7, E = 7 for 400 stories; p = NS). The focus of the story is, for example, that one person uses the second to obtain money, sex, work, or information.

Two qualities of an interaction which provide one possible complement to relations seen as asymmetric or exploitatory involve mutuality and empathy. A count of instances where mutuality, cooperation, and commonality are the focal theme of a story shows this is more typically an *E*'s story (I = 7, E = 25 for 300 stories; p < .01. I = 21, E = 33 for 400 stories; p = .11). An operation for scoring empathy, defined as an expression of concern of one person for the suffering, injury, or hardship of a second, yields similar results. *E*s are more likely to describe one person "feeling for" the plight of another (I = 4, E = 16 for 300 stories; p < .01. I = 5, E = 10 for 400 stories; p = .28).

Appendix C. Data and Distribution of Subjects: TAT Project

Table 2. Sex × I/E designation of two pools of subjects.

| | First pool | | | Second pool | | | Combined pools | |
	I	E		I	E		I	E
Male	8	9	Male	16	16	Male	24	25
Female	7	6	Female	14	14	Female	21	20
Total	15	15	Total	30	30	Total	45	45

Table 3. Rules and dimensions.

			Criterion				
			I	E			
		Score I	A	B			
Rule or dimension		No score	C	D			
Rule	A	B	C	D	N	$\chi^{2\,a}$	P
1	15	3	30	42	90	8.4	< .01
2	10	2	35	43	90	4.7	< .03
3	24	9	21	36	90	9.3	< .01
4	17	5	28	40	90	7.2	< .01
5	30	9	15	36	90	18.1	< .01
6	32	12	13	33	90	16.0	< .01
7	18	6	27	39	90	6.8	< .01
Dimension[b]							
Distance (first definition)	22	7	128	143	300	7.4	< .01
Distance (expanded definition)	59	32	131	118	400	9.6	< .01
Distance (expanded definition)	111	54	339	396	900	23.3	< .01
N Aff	20	31	130	119	300	2.4	.14
"No-relation"	11	7	139	143	300	–	NS
N Ach	14	11	86	89	200	–	NS
N Pow	10	8	90	92	200	–	NS
Action toward	12	21	138	129	300	2.1	.15
Action toward	18	22	182	178	400	–	NS
Action toward (mutual)	3	11	147	139	300	3.6	.06
Action toward (mutual)	14	24	186	176	400	2.1	.15
Action away	13	7	137	143	300	1.3	.25
Action away	15	18	185	183	400	–	NS
Action against	35	30	115	120	300	–	NS

Table 3. (Continued)

Dimension	A	B	Score I No score C	Criterion I A E B C D	N	χ^{2} [a]	P
Action against (within relation)	25	12	125	138	300	3.7	.06
Action against (within relation)	28	21	172	179	400	–	NS
Internal punishment	10	16	140	136	300	1.05	NS
Internal punishment	7	14	193	186	400	1.8	.19
Asymmetry	11	4	139	146	300	2.5	.12
Asymmetry	22	15	178	185	400	–	NS
Action against (exploitation)	13	5	137	145	300	2.9	.09
Action against (exploitation)	7	7	193	193	400	–	NS
Mutuality	7	25	143	125	300	10.1	< .01
Mutuality	21	33	179	167	400	2.6	.11
Empathy	4	16	146	134	300	3.9	.05
Empathy	5	10	195	190	400	1.1	.28
Self-concern	20	5	130	145	300	8.5	< .01
Self-concern	13	7	187	193	400	1.3	.25

[a]All χ^2s have *df* = 1.

[b]Some of the responses in this section of the χ^2 tables come from the same subjects. Therefore, these responses may not be uncorrelated, as the assumptions of the test require. However, although the χ^2s may be inflated as a result of possible correlational contamination, and while the precision of the test is diminished, it is felt that the exploratory nature and the heuristic value of these findings allow their acceptability in this context. The data used in the derivation of the seven "I" rules do, of course, meet the independence requirements of the χ^2 test.

Table 4. Affect operations.[a]

Cards	Affect words	Criterion I	E	
One Figure	Neg.	30	30	$\chi^2 = 1.3, p = .23, df = 1$
	Pos.	22	12	
	194			
"Many" Figures	Neg.	8	3	$\chi^2 = 2.2, p = .14, df = 1$
	Pos.	4	6	
	121			

Table 4. (Continued)

Cards	Affect words	Criterion		
		I	E	
Two Figures	Neg.	20	9	χ^2 = 4.8, p = .03, df = 1
	Pos.	6	13	
		148		
Across Cards	Neg.	58	32	χ^2 = 2.5, p = .12, df = 1
	Pos.	32	31	
		153		

[a] As in the "dimensions" in Table 3, these responses are not uncorrelated.

Table 5. Overlapping and nonoverlapping instances of each of three pairs of rules drawn from the same card, for combined pools (N = 90).

		Criterion	
		I	E
Rules 1 and 2:	1 only	11	4
	2 only	6	1
	both	4	0
Rules 3 and 4:	3 only	17	8
	4 only	10	4
	both	7	1
Rules 5 and 6:	5 only	7	3
	6 only	9	6
	both	23	6

Table 6. Ratios of agreement to disagreement of seven "I" rules, by sex

Rule	Male[a] criterion		Female criterion	
	I	E	I	E
1	8	1	7	2
2	5	2	5	0
3	13	5	11	4
4	9	3	8	2
5	15	6	15	3
6	16	8	16	4
7	10	1	8	5

[a]Note that there are 49 males and 41 females in the combined pools.

References

Allport, G. W. *Becoming: Basic considerations for a psychology of personality.* New Haven: Yale Univ. Press, 1955.

Atkinson, J. W. (Ed.), *Motives in fantasy, action, and society.* Princeton, N.J.: Van Nostrand, 1958.

Atkinson, J. W., Heyns, R. W., and Veroff, J. The effect of experimental arousal of the affiliation motive on thematic apperception. *Journal of Abnormal and Social Psychology,* 1954, **49**, 405–410.

Bakan, P., Belton, J. A., and Toth, J. C. Extraversion-introversion and decrement in an auditory vigilance task. In P. Bakan (Ed.), *Attention.* Princeton, N.J.: Van Nostrand, 1966.

Baldwin, A. L. *Theories of child development.* New York: Wiley, 1968.

Bash, K. W. Einstellungstypus and Erlebnistypus: C. G. Jung and Herman Rorschach. *Journal of Projective Techniques,* 1955, **19**, 236–242.

Bennett, E. A. *What Jung really said.* New York: Schocken Books, 1967.

Bieler, S. H. Some correlates of the Jungian typology: Personal style variables. Master's thesis, Duke University, 1966.

Bleibtreu, J. *The parable of the beast.* Toronto: Collier Books, 1968.

Boss, M. *Psychoanalysis and Daseinanalysis.* New York: Basic Books, 1963.

Bradway, K. Jung's psychological types. *Journal of Analytical Psychology,* 1964, **9**, 130–140.

Bruner, J. S., and Goodman, C. C. Value and need as organizing factors in perception. *Journal of Abnormal and Social Psychology,* 1947, **42**, 33–44.

Buber, M. *Between man and man.* Boston: Beacon Press, 1955.

Buber, M. *I and thou.* New York: Scribners, 1958.

Buckley, F. An approach to a phenomenology of at-homeness. In A. Giorgi et al. (Eds.), *Duquesne studies in phenomenological psychology,* vol. 1. Pittsburgh: Duquesne Univ. Press, 1971.

Bugental, J. *The search for authenticity.* New York: Holt, Rinehart and Winston, 1965.

Carrigan, P. M. Extraversion-introversion as a dimension of personality: A reappraisal. *Psychological Bulletin,* 1960, **57**, 329–360.

Chein, I. *Science of behavior and the image of man.* New York: Basic Books, 1972.

Colaizzi, P. F. Analysis of the learner's perception of learning material at various phases of a learning process. In A. Giorgi et al. (Eds.), *Duquesne studies in phenomenological psychology,* vol. 1. Pittsburgh: Duquesne Univ. Press, 1971.

Combs, A., and Snygg, D. *Individual behavior: A perceptual approach to behavior.* New York: Harper and Row, 1959.

Cook, D. Is Jung's typology true? Unpublished doctoral dissertation, Duke University, 1970.

Copleston, F. *A history of philosophy,* vol. 4. Garden City, N.Y.: Doubleday, 1963.

Dicks-Mireaux, M. J. Extraversion-introversion in experimental psychology: Examples of experimental evidence and their theoretical implications. *Journal of Analytical Psychology,* 1964, **9**, 117–129.

Edwards, A. L. *Statistical methods for the behavioral sciences.* New York: Holt, Rinehart, and Winston, 1964.

Eysenck, H. J. Cortical inhibition, figural after-effect, and personality. *Journal of Abnormal and Social Psychology,* 1955, **51**, 94–106.

Eysenck, H. J. *The biological basis of personality.* Springfield, Ill.: Charles C. Thomas, 1967.

Eysenck, H. J., and Rachman, S. Dimensions of personality. In B. Semeonoff (Ed.), *Personality assessment.* Baltimore: Penguin Books, 1966.

Eysenck, Sybil B., and Eysenck, H. J. On the dual nature of extraversion. *British Journal of Social and Clinical Psychology,* 1963, **2**, 46–55.

Farber, Leslie. *The ways of the will.* New York: Basic Books, 1966.

Farber, M. *Phenomenology and existence.* New York: Harper and Row, 1967.

Fischer, C. Toward the structure of privacy: Implications for psychological assessment. In A. Giorgi et al. (Eds.), *Duquesne studies in phenomenological psychology,* vol. 1. Pittsburgh: Duquesne Univ. Press, 1971.

Flavell, J. H. *The developmental psychology of Jean Piaget.* Princeton, N.J.: Van Nostrand, 1963.

Fordham, F. *An introduction to Jung's psychology.* Baltimore: Penguin Books, 1956.

Gendlin, E. T. *Experiencing and the creation of meaning.* Toronto: Free Press of Glencoe, 1962.

Gendlin, E. T. Experiential explication and truth. *Journal of Existentialism,* 1966, **6**, 131–146.

Gendlin, E. T. Focusing. *Psychotherapy: Theory, research, and practice,* 1969, **6**, 4–15.

Giorgi, A., et al. (Eds.), *Duquesne studies in phenomenological psychology,* vol. 1. Pittsburgh: Duquesne Univ. Press, 1971.

Gore, M. P., and Rotter, J. B. A personality correlate of social action. *Journal of Personality,* 1963, **31**, 58–64.

Gorlow, L., Simonson, N. R., and Krauss, H. An empirical investigation of the Jungian typology. *British Journal of Social and Clinical Psychology,* 1966, **5**, 108–117.

Gough, H. G. *California personality inventory manual.* Palo Alto, Calif.: Consulting Psychologists' Press, 1964.

Gray, H., and Wheelwright, J. B. Jung's psychological types, their frequency of occurrence. *Journal of General Psychology,* 1946, **34**, 3–17.

Grinker, R. *The borderline syndrome.* New York: Basic Books, 1968.

Guilford, J. P. *An inventory of factors STDCR.* Beverly Hills, Calif.: Sheridan Supply Co., 1940.

Guilford, J. P., and Braly, K. W. Extraversion and introversion. *Psychological Bulletin,* 1930, **27**, 96–107.

Hart, J., and Tomlinson, T. (Eds.), *New directions in client-centered psychotherapy.* Boston: Houghton-Mifflin, 1970.

Heidegger, M. *Being and time.* New York: Harper and Row, 1962.

Heidegger, M. *Existence and being.* Chicago: Henry Regnery, 1970.

Heisenberg, W. *Physics and beyond: Encounters and conversations.* New York: Harper Torchbooks, 1972.

Henry, W. E. *The analysis of fantasy.* New York: Wiley, 1956.

Hesse, H. *Siddhartha.* Binghamton, N.Y.: New Directions, 1957.

Hesse, H. *Demian.* New York: Bantam Books, 1968.

Horney, Karen. *Neurotic personality of our time.* New York: Norton, 1937.

Husserl, E. *Cartesian meditations. An introduction to phenomenology.* The Hague: Martinus Nijhoff, 1970.

Husserl, E. *Paris lectures.* The Hague: Martinus Nijhoff, 1970.

Jacobi, Jolande. *The psychology of C. G. Jung.* New Haven: Yale Univ. Press, 1962.

James, W. *Psychology: The briefer course.* New York: Harper and Brothers, 1961.

Jung, C. G. On psychical energy. In *Contributions to analytical psychology.* Trans. by C. F. and H. G. Baynes. New York: Harcourt, Brace, 1928.

Jung, C. G. *Psychological types.* Trans. by H. G. Baynes. London: Routledge and Kegan Paul, 1923.

Jung, C. G. *Two essays on analytical psychology.* Trans. by R. F. C. Hull. New York: World Book, 1953.

Jung, C. G. *Psyche and symbol.* Garden City, N.Y.: Doubleday, 1958.

Jung, C. G. *Memories, dreams, reflections.* Trans. by Richard and Clara Winston. New York: Vintage Books, 1965.

Jung, C. G. *Analytical psychology: Its theory and practice.* New York: Pantheon Books, 1968.

Jung, C. G. (Ed.), *Man and his symbols.* Garden City, N.Y.: Doubleday, 1969.

Kagan, J. Reflection-impulsivity: The generality and dynamics of conceptual tempo. *Journal of Abnormal Psychology,* 1966, 71, 17–24.

Kaufmann, W. *Hegel: Reinterpretation and commentary.* Garden City, N.Y.: Doubleday, 1965.

Kelly, G. A. *A theory of personality: The psychology of personal constructs.* New York: W. W. Norton, 1963.

Koch, S. Psychology and emerging conceptions of knowledge as unitary. In T. W. Wann (Ed.), *Behaviorism and phenomenology.* Chicago: Univ. of Chicago Press, 1964.

Kockelmans, J. (Ed.), *Phenomenology: The philosophy of Edmund Husserl and its interpretations.* Garden City, N.Y.: Doubleday, 1967.

Koestler, A. *The ghost in the machine.* Chicago: Henry Regnery, 1967.

Laing, R. D. *The divided self.* Baltimore: Pelican, 1965.

Lecky, P. *Self-consistency: A theory of personality.* Garden City, N.Y.: Doubleday, 1969.

Lewin, K. *A dynamic theory of personality.* New York: McGraw-Hill, 1935.

Linschoten, H. *On the way toward a phenomenological psychology: The psychology of William James.* Pittsburgh: Duquesne Univ. Press, 1968.

Luijpen, W. *Existential phenomenology.* Pittsburgh: Duquesne Univ. Press, 1969.

MacLeod, R. B. Phenomenology: A challenge to experimental psychology. In T. W. Wann (Ed.), *Behaviorism and phenomenology*. Chicago: University of Chicago Press, 1964.

Marshall, I. N. Extraversion and libido in Jung and Cattell. *Journal of Analytical Psychology*, 1967, **12**, 115–136.

Maslow, A. *Toward a psychology of being*. Princeton, N.J.: Van Nostrand, 1962.

Matson, F. *The broken image*. New York: Braziller, 1964.

May, R. *Love and will*. New York: Norton, 1969.

May, R. (Ed.), *Existential psychology*. New York: Random House, 1961.

May, R., Angel, E., and Ellenberger, H. F. (Eds.), *Existence: A new dimension in psychiatry and psychology*. New York: Basic Books, 1958.

McClelland, D. C. Measuring motivation in phantasy. In R. C. Birney and R. C. Teevan (Eds.), *Measuring human motivation*. Princeton, N.J.: Van Nostrand, 1962.

McClelland, D. C., Atkinson, J. W., Clark, R. A., and Lowell, E. C. *The achievement motive*. New York: Appleton-Century-Crofts 1953.

Merleau-Ponty, M. *Phenomenology of perception*. New York: Humanities, 1962.

Merleau-Ponty, M. *The structure of behavior*. Trans. by A. L. Fisher. Boston: Beacon Press, 1963.

Moustakas, C. *Loneliness*. Englewood Cliffs, N. J.: Prentice-Hall, 1961.

Murray, H. A. *Explorations in personality*. New York: Oxford Univ. Press, 1938.

Murray, H. Techniques for a systematic investigation of fantasy. *Journal of Psychology*, 1936, **3**, 115–143.

Murray, H. *Thematic Apperception Test Manual*. Cambridge, Mass.: Harvard College, 1943.

Murstein, B. (Ed.), *Handbook of projective techniques*. New York: Basic Books, 1965.

Myers, Isabel B. *The Myers-Briggs Type Indicator: Manual*. Princeton, N.J.: Educational Testing Service, 1962.

Natanson, M. *The journeying self: A study in philosophy and social role*. Reading, Mass.: Addison-Wesley, 1970.

Perls, F. *Gestalt therapy verbatim*. Lafayette, Calif.: Real People Press, 1969.

Polanyi, M. *The tacit dimension*. Garden City, N.Y.: Doubleday, 1966.

Purcell, K. The TAT and antisocial behavior. In B. Murstein (Ed.), *Handbook of projective techniques*. New York: Basic Books, 1965.

Riesman, D. *The lonely crowd*. New Haven: Yale Univ. Press, 1963.

Rogers, C. R. *Client-centered therapy*. Boston: Houghton-Mifflin, 1965.

Rokeach, M. *The open and closed mind*. New York: Basic Books, 1960.

Romanyshyn, R. An empirical investigation of the experience of anger. In A. Giorgi et al. (Eds.), *Duquesne studies in phenomenological psychology*, vol. 1. Pittsburgh: Duquesne Univ. Press, 1971.

Ruitenbeek, H. (Ed.), *Psychoanalysis and existential philosophy*. New York: E. P. Dutton, 1962.

Sadler, W. A. *Existence and love: A new approach to existential phenomenology*. New York: Scribners, 1969.

Sartre, J. *Being and nothingness*. New York: Washington Square Press, 1966.

Schachtel, E. *Metamorphosis: On the development of affect, perception, attention, and memory.* New York: Basic Books, 1959.

Schachtel, E. G. *Experiential foundations of Rorschach's test.* New York: Basic Books, 1966.

Schachter, S. *Psychology of affiliation.* Stanford: Stanford University Press, 1959.

Serrano, M. *C. G. Jung and Hermann Hesse: A record of two friendships* (Trans. by F. MacShane). New York: Schocken Books, 1966.

Severin, F. (Ed.), *Humanistic viewpoints in psychology.* New York: McGraw-Hill, 1965.

Shapiro, K. J. A critique of introversion. *Spring: An annual of archetypal psychology and Jungian thought,* 1972, 60–74.

Shapiro, K. J. The concept of introversion. Unpublished doctoral dissertation, Duke University, 1971.

Shapiro, K. J., and Alexander, I. E. Extraversion-introversion, affiliation, and anxiety. *Journal of Personality,* 1969, 37, 387–406.

Shipley, T. E., and Veroff, J. A projective measure of need for affiliation. In R. C. Birney and R. C. Teevan (Eds.), *Measuring human motivation.* Princeton, N.J.: Van Nostrand, 1962.

Shlien, J. (Ed.), *Research in psychotherapy,* vol. 3. American Psychological Association, Washington, D.C., 1967.

Singer, J. L. *Daydreaming, an introduction to the experimental study of inner experience.* New York: Random House, 1966.

Snow, C. P. *The two cultures and the scientific revolution.* New York: Cambridge Univ. Press, 1960.

Snygg, D., and Combs, A. *Individual behavior: A new frame of reference for psychology.* New York: Harper and Row, 1949.

Sonneman, U. *Existence and therapy: An introduction to phenomenological psychology and existential analysis.* New York: Grune and Stratton, 1954.

Spiegelberg, H. *The Phenomenological Movement: A historical introduction,* vols. 1 and 2. The Hague: Martinus Nijhoff, 1969.

Stanfiel, J. D. The typological approach in personality. Unpublished paper, Duke University, 1964.

Stevick, E. Toward a phenomenology of attitudes. In A. Giorgi et al. (Eds.), *Duquesne studies in phenomenological psychology,* vol. 1. Pittsburgh: Duquesne Univ. Press, 1971.

Storms, L. H., and Sigal, J. J. Eysenck's personality theory. *British Journal of Medical Psychology,* 1958, 31, 228–246.

Straus, E. W. *Phenomenological psychology.* London: Tavistock, 1966.

Stricker, L. J., and Ross, J. An assessment of some of the structural properties of the Jungian typology. *Journal of Abnormal and Social Psychology,* 1964, 68, 62–71.

Tart, C. (Ed.), *Altered states of consciousness.* New York: Wiley, 1969.

Teilhard de Chardin, P. *The phenomenon of man.* New York: Harper and Brothers, 1959.

Van den Berg, J. H. *The phenomenological approach to psychiatry.* Springfield, Ill.: Charles C Thomas, 1955.

Van den Berg, J. H. *Changing nature of man.* New York: Norton, 1961.

Van Kaam, A. Phenomenal analysis: Exemplified by a study of the experience of 'really feeling understood.' *Journal of Individual Psychology,* 1959, **15**, 66–72.

Van Kaam, A. *Existential foundations of psychology.* Pittsburgh: Duquesne Univ. Press, 1966.

Veroff, J. Development and validation of a projective measure of power motivation. *Journal of Abnormal and Social Psychology,* 1957, **54**, 1–8.

von Franz, M., and Hillman, J. *Lectures on Jung's typology.* New York: Spring Publications, 1971.

von Uexkuell, J. J. A stroll through the worlds of animals and men. In Claire Schiller (Ed.), *Instinctive behavior.* New York: International Universities Press, 1957.

Wallach, M. *Modes of thinking in young children.* New York: Holt, Rinehart and Winston, 1965.

Wallach, M. Thinking, feeling, and expressing: Toward understanding the person. In R. Jessor and S. Feshbach (Eds.), *Cognition, personality, and clinical psychology.* San Francisco: Jossey-Bass, 1967.

Wallach, M. A., and Gahm, R. C. Personality functions of graphic constriction and expansiveness. *Journal of Personality,* 1960, **28**, 73–88.

Wann, T. W. (Ed.), *Behaviorism and phenomenology.* Chicago: Univ. of Chicago Press, 1964.

Watts, A. *Psychotherapy east and west.* New York: New American Library, 1963.

Webster's seventh new collegiate dictionary. Springfield, Mass.: G. C. Merriam Co., 1963.

Witkin, H. A., Dyk, R. B., Faterson, H. F., Goodenough, D. R., and Karp, S. A. *Psychological differentiation.* New York: Wiley, 1962.

Index

Abstraction, 148
Activism, and I/E differences, 140–41
Activity, introversion and, 16, 17, 145
Adaptation, 47
Adler, Alfred, 22–23, 115
Affect, 67–68, 151, 162; TAT data on, 169–70
Affiliation, 65–67, 73–75, 78, 106–107, 145, 150–51
Aggression, tendency toward, 66–67, 166
Alienation, 158
Anxiety, 73–75
Archetypal figures, 38
Atkinson, J. W., 65, 66
Attitude, Jung on, 18, 54, 75, 115
Autia, 16
Autism, 70
Autonomy, 69. *See also* Self-reliance

Behavior, prediction of, 74, 76, 78
Bennett, E. A., 22–23
Bias, 84–85, 86, 110
Bieler, S. H., 150, 167
Blame, placing of, 67, 150, 167
Boss, Medard, 92, 93, 94
Buber, Martin, 5, 93, 95

Carrigan, P. M., 12, 15, 16
Cartesianism, 89, 94, 110, 114, 115
Colaizzi, P. F., 107, 108
Collective unconscious, 25–31 *passim*, 40, 41, 48; emergence and, 144; self and, 46
Consciousness, 5, 91; Jung on, 115, 124–25; subjective and objective determinants of, 125, 128. *See also* Perception
Control, sense of, 140–41
Culture, 25, 29, 45–46, 47, 53, 85

Definition, problem of, 81
Depression, 16, 67, 165
Descartes, René, 89, 90. *See also* Cartesianism
Distance, interpersonal, 60, 61–64, 67, 70, 74, 75, 119, 129, 135–36, 156–58, 159; TAT data on, 168
Dominance, 38; and I/E differences, 16, 66, 167
Dualism, 89–90, 91, 94, 95, 114, 115. *See also* Opposites; Polarity

Ectopsyche, 41, 42
Ego, 90; and introversion, 45–46, 49; and

neurotic guilt, 149; "transcendental," 104. *See also* Self
Emergence, theme of, 143–45
Empathy, 10, 159–60, 167, 169
Empirical data, 102–103, 106–108, 110–11, 144, 147–48. *See also* Thematic Apperception Test
Enantiodromia, 39
Encounter, 5, 8; experience as, 126–27, 148; and I/E difference, 152, 153–56, 157, 159
Encounter movement, 7
Endopsyche, 41, 42, 43
Energy, 32–37, 42, 47. *See also* Libido
Epistemology, 6–7, 9
Ethology, 8
Existence, phenomenological concept of, 94
Existential therapy, 7, 92, 97, 102
Existentialism, 5, 6
Experience: antinomies in, 114, 116; lived and reflected, relation between, 94–103, 104, 111–12, 113–14, 116, 131; phenomenology and, 83, 87–92, 104; and problem of I/E, 116–27; reflected, 130–34, 145–46, 153–57; relational nature of, 92–94; and self, 137–42, 150; shared vs. unique, 119–20, 125–27, 142, 143, 153, 155–56, 161; validity of empirical data on, 102–103, 106, 112–113, 133
Experiencing and the Creation of Meaning (Gendlin), 131
Explication, 98, 100, 102
Extraversion, 14, 16, 22, 23, 26–27, 33, 47; affiliative tendencies, 65–67; experience of, 120–21; and intimacy, 160–61; Jung on, 29–30, 35, 41, 78–79; and reflected experience, 132–34, 137–38; and testing methods, 54, 78; view of self, 139–43. *See also* Introversion-extraversion
Eysenck, H. J., 16n

Farber, Leslie, 81, 88
"Felt-meaning," 11, 96–97, 98–103, 104–105, 111, 131
Fischer, C., 108–109
Freud, Sigmund, 20, 22, 32–33, 41, 115

Gendlin, Eugene, 3, 5, 7, 8, 9, 80, 89, 113; on "felt-meaning," 11, 95–103 *passim*, 131
Goldstein, K., 148
Gorlow, L., 53–54

178